the 30-minute
diabetes
cookbook

azmina govindji

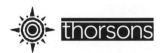

Thorsons
An Imprint of HarperCollins*Publishers*
77–85 Fulham Palace Road,
Hammersmith, London W6 8JB

The website address is: www.thorsonselement.com

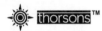

and *Thorsons* are trademarks of
HarperCollins*Publishers* Ltd

Some of the recipes in this volume have been published
previously in *Quick and Easy Cooking for Diabetes*
This revised and updated version published by Thorsons 2003

10 9 8 7 6 5 4 3 2 1

A catalogue record of this book
is available from the British Library

ISBN 0 00 714971 9

Printed and bound in Great Britain by
Martins the Printers, Berwick upon Tweed

Contents

Acknowledgements

Such a comprehensive and tasty collection of recipes doesn't come easy. I must thank my colleagues, Elaine Gardner and Marilyn Cunningham, for helping me add diversity to the dishes, and life coach Nina Puddefoot for giving me the inspiration to write the motivational tips in the Introduction. I'd also like to thank Diabetes UK for reading the manuscript. And, as always, family support is crucial when I'm writing a new book, and Shamil, Bizhan and Shazia have been an absolute dream!

Introduction

Whether you've been diagnosed with diabetes or care for someone with the condition, the facts and ideas in this book are likely to leave you feeling uplifted. Why? The way you see diabetes, the way you feel about having the condition (including the 'why me?' factor), and how you make food choices will all influence the way you deal with day-to-day situations. By taking some simple steps, both practical and through positive thinking, you can enjoy life without letting diabetes overwhelm you.

What is Diabetes?

When you have diabetes, the amount of glucose (sugar) in your blood is too high because your body cannot use it properly. Glucose comes mainly from the digestion of starchy foods such as bread and potatoes, and sweet foods like sweets and chocolates. A hormone called insulin helps glucose enter the cells where it is used as fuel by the body. If there is not enough insulin, or if the insulin you have is not working well, then glucose can build up in your blood. This causes the classic symptoms of diabetes:

- thirst and a dry mouth
- passing large amounts of urine (especially at night)
- loss of weight
- tiredness
- genital itchiness
- blurring of vision

If you think about it more closely, when glucose cannot get into the cells, you are unable to use it for energy and daily activity. The consequence of not 'moving' the glucose into the cells is that the glucose builds up in your blood. This leads to the long-term complications of diabetes such as heart disease, nerve damage, kidney disease and vision impairment. If you have diabetes, you already have an increased risk of developing heart disease, so watching what you eat is particularly important. And that is where this cookbook can make a big difference.

Types of Diabetes

There is no cure for diabetes, and there is no such thing as mild diabetes. However, with the appropriate treatment and a healthy attitude, you can enjoy a full and active life. There are two main types of diabetes.

Type 1 Diabetes (or Insulin Dependent Diabetes)

This occurs when the body has a severe shortage of its own insulin. It is treated by insulin injections and a healthy way of eating based on regular meals and snacks. It usually occurs in people under 40 years of age. People who require insulin as medication will need to take it in the form of an injection since, if taken by mouth, it would be digested in the gut. There are many different types of insulin, with different actions in the body, and your diabetes specialist will work with you to find the best combination.

Type 2 Diabetes (or Non-insulin Dependent Diabetes)

This is the most common type of diabetes. About 75 per cent of people with diabetes are not dependent on insulin. Here, the body can still make some insulin, but not enough for its needs. People with Type 2 diabetes are usually overweight and are advised to reduce weight by eating a range of healthy foods. Some people may also need tablets. This condition usually affects people over about 40 years of age but, with rising rates of obesity, more and more Type 2 diabetes is being diagnosed at a younger age.

Some people *require* insulin to treat their diabetes but are not truly insulin-dependent. They may be treated by following a healthy diet, tablets and insulin injections.

Insulin or tablets are not a substitute for healthy meals.

Get in the Know...

There is an old saying – ignorance is bliss. Not so! Ignorance carries a price that could have direct consequences on your health and, in particular, your diabetes. If you make choices from some of the guidelines in this book, you are demonstrating responsibility and accountability for your own life. This is very important if you want to remain in control of your world. After all, you are running your own show.

There may well be people in your life who will happily tell you what you should and shouldn't do, but that may mean you will carry on without truly making choices for yourself. If you do what you've always done, you'll get what you've always got! Compare this to someone who takes total accountability for the results and consequences of their choices. If they take the initiative and action to do something different, they will at some stage reap the fruits of their labour.

The prospect of 'driving your own bus', so to speak, can feel quite scary, but that is how you achieve true control over your life. If, as you read this, it dawns on you that perhaps you could do more for yourself (which might simply be caring for your diabetes), then choose to do it, today. Many people continue through their life's journey, content to have their bus driven. This keeps them 'safe' as there will always be someone else to blame, a reason or excuse for things not working out.

Perhaps you could put yourself back in the driving seat by learning and understanding the facts that surround this condition so you can treat your diabetes more effectively. There is access to so much information – how can you use it to empower yourself? You could make a list of ideas right now. You may come up with several you either haven't thought of before or haven't yet acted on. Try to keep an open and flexible mind.

What's so Important about Food?

Food plays an integral role in helping to regulate your blood glucose levels, because what you eat and how often can have a significant effect on blood glucose. There is no such thing as a special diabetic diet. A range of healthy foods such as the dishes in this book can be beneficial whether you have diabetes or not. As each person varies in their dietary requirements, it is recommended that people diagnosed with diabetes visit a state-registered dietitian for tailored dietary advice.

Eating well can influence your blood glucose levels, blood pressure, blood cholesterol, blood triglycerides and your weight. A healthy balance of meals and snacks can have lasting effects on your long-term health and can give you that 'feel-good factor' too!

Making the Right Food Choices

- Eat regular meals.
- Choose starchy foods that contain complex carbohydrates (such as wholegrain bread, pasta and porridge, *see below*).
- Regularly eat foods with a low glycaemic load (such as beans, peas, lentils, vegetables, fruit and oats, *see opposite*).
- Watch your intake of fried and fatty foods (such as butter, full-fat cheese, fatty meats, crisps and pastries, *see pages 6–7*).
- Eat five portions of fruit and vegetables a day (*see opposite*).
- Swap high-sugar foods (such as tinned fruit in syrup, sugared drinks) for low-sugar foods (such as tinned fruit in natural juice, sugar-free drinks, *see page 7*).
- Eat a portion of oily fish once a week. Research suggests that this can significantly reduce the incidence of heart disease, and it even benefits people who have already suffered a heart attack.
- Keep an eye on how much salt you use. A high salt intake is linked with high blood pressure. Use other flavourings such as herbs and spices instead.
- Limit the amount of alcohol you drink (*see page 12*).

There are lots of healthy-eating tips in this book. It's a good idea to pick out the changes you feel will fit easily into your lifestyle, choosing foods you enjoy. And there's no need to think there are foods you *must* eat and those you must not. Healthy eating is all about balance – choosing a variety of healthy foods you enjoy and not forcing yourself to eat foods you dislike. By flicking through the pages in this book, you'll see that there are choices for everyone.

Below are some suggestions on how you can include healthier items on your menu. You may find that you already choose many of the recommended foods, so eating well may be easier than you think.

Starchy Foods

Starchy carbohydrate foods such as bread, rice, pasta, cereals, chapatis and potatoes are naturally low in fat and can help to fill you up. Cutting down on meat and cheese portions and basing meals on starchy, lower-fat foods instead can be helpful if you're trying to lose weight.

Wholegrain varieties of bread and cereals as well as the skin on potatoes are high in fibre. High-fibre starchy foods, such as bran-based cereals and wholemeal bread, are especially useful in preventing constipation. A high-fibre diet is recommended for the whole family, but remember that when you eat more fibre, it is important to drink more fluid. Try to have at least six to eight cups of fluid (such as water or low-calorie drinks) each day.

Oat-based cereals like porridge and muesli are high in a particular type of fibre called soluble fibre. These foods are absorbed even more slowly than starchy foods in general, and they can play a significant part in keeping your blood glucose within a healthy range. Instant hot oats cereals do contain soluble fibre, but because the oats have been 'mashed up', they have less effect on slowing down the rise in blood glucose after meals (see 'Glycaemic Index', page 7).

It is important to spread your intake of starchy foods evenly throughout the day and to eat regular meals. This helps to reduce fluctuations in your blood glucose levels.

Fruit and Vegetables

These foods contain important vitamins that are needed for health, whether you have diabetes or not. A diet containing plenty of fruit and vegetables will provide more fibre, especially soluble fibre, more antioxidant vitamins and will usually be lower in fat. The antioxidant vitamins – betacarotene (which is converted to vitamin A in the body), vitamins C and E – have been linked to a lower incidence of heart disease, some cancers and gut problems.

For good health, it is recommended that you eat five portions of fruit and vegetables (not counting potatoes) daily. There's no need to buy fresh vegetables if you haven't got time to prepare them. Frozen varieties are just as nutritious. Try to cook them quickly in the minimum amount of boiling water, or better still, steam them and serve immediately. This helps to preserve much of the vitamin content.

To keep your fat intake down, avoid adding butter or margarine to cooked vegetables. If you need a dressing on salads, try a fat-free vinaigrette or simply use some lemon juice or low-fat natural yoghurt. Flavour this with coarsely ground black pepper and fresh or dried herbs to your taste.

Drinking large amounts of fruit juice, even if this is unsweetened, can make your blood glucose rise sharply. This is because the natural sugar in a liquid form is rapidly absorbed by the body. If you like fresh fruit juice, take it with a meal rather than on its own. Alternatively, choose a sugar-free squash, diet drink or water.

Vitamin supplements alone are not a replacement for fruit and vegetables.

Fats and Oils

One of the key tips for eating well, whether you have diabetes or not, is to keep an eye on the fatty foods you eat. Saturated fat, found in meat and dairy products, has been shown to raise a type of fat in your blood called cholesterol. High blood cholesterol makes you more prone to heart problems. Since people with diabetes are at an increased risk of getting heart disease, watching your fat intake is particularly important. Foods high in saturated fat include full-fat milk and cheese, fatty meat, lard, dripping, sausages, pies and pastries.

Replace some of the foods that contain a lot of saturated fat with those high in monounsaturated or polyunsaturated fat. For example, use small amounts of rapeseed, olive, corn or sunflower oil in cooking and spread butter or margarine sparingly. There is now a wide variety of lower-fat foods available in supermarkets. Use reduced-fat versions of dairy products, such as semi-skimmed or skimmed milk, half-fat cheddar cheese and low-fat yoghurt. Note that reduced-fat products can only help you cut down on fat and calories as long as you don't eat twice as much!

Trans fats are hydrogenated oils or fats that can raise your blood cholesterol levels, so are best eaten in limited amounts. They are often found in spreads and margarines, biscuits, pies, cakes and pastries.

Meat, Fish, Nuts, Pulses and Eggs

These foods are rich in protein and many are good sources of vitamins and minerals, such as iron and zinc. However, since meat can be high in saturated fat, it is best to choose lean cuts and to minimize the oil you use in cooking. Here are some tips on choosing healthy foods from this group.

- Select lean cuts of meat and trim off visible fat. Try to cook meat without adding fat by grilling (broiling), roasting (as in 'Lamb cutlets with tomato and mint sauce', *page 47*) and braising. Avoid using the juices from roast meat for gravy.
- Remove the skin from poultry.
- Grill meat products such as sausages and burgers and allow the fat to drain off.
- Eat oily fish once a week, such as salmon, herring and mackerel (try 'Turkish mackerel wraps', *page 84*).
- Nuts are an important source of protein if you are vegetarian. Recent research suggests that eating an ounce (about a handful) of nuts such as peanuts and

almonds a day may help protect against heart disease, but they are also high in fat, so avoid eating too many.

- Pulses such as beans, sweetcorn, peas and lentils are an excellent source of soluble fibre. Choose them regularly. They are cheap and nutritious and can make main meals go further (as in 'Chilli con carne', *page 126*).
- Eggs can be poached, boiled or scrambled instead of fried.
- If you rely on lots of convenience foods, look out for lower-fat and lower-salt versions of ready meals.

Sugar and Sweet Foods

You do not have to avoid sugar completely. The effect of food on your blood glucose does not depend only on sugar content, but on a whole range of other factors such as how the food is cooked and what is eaten with it. Small amounts of sugar, when taken as part of a meal, do not have a detrimental effect on your blood glucose levels. Only drinks and foods that have sugar as the main ingredient are best avoided, as they can make your blood glucose rise sharply, particularly if they are taken on their own between meals. Use reduced amounts of sugar in baking and desserts and replace with fresh or dried fruit for sweetness.

Glycaemic Index (GI)

The GI is a ranking of foods, which relates to how they affect blood glucose levels. The faster a food is broken down during digestion, the quicker will be the rise in blood glucose. Since one of the main aims of treating diabetes is to keep blood glucose levels steady throughout the day, foods which cause sharp rises in blood glucose are best kept to a minimum (unless needed for special circumstances, such as illness, hypoglycaemia or exercise). Foods that cause a rapid rise in blood glucose will have a high GI or a high glycaemic load, so the key is to choose more foods with a lower glycaemic load regularly.

A lot of this will be common sense: 'whole' foods, such as whole grains, and those high in 'soluble fibre', such as kidney beans, will take longer to be broken down by the body and will thus cause a slower rise in blood glucose. If you imagine how easy it is to digest some hummus – it's already in small particles (and quite sloppy, though delicious!) – it would make sense to suggest that the body doesn't need to mash this up for too long before the hummus is digested and ready to go into the bloodstream as glucose.

Now imagine how much longer it would take for you to digest a whole chickpea casserole. The body needs to break down the skin before it even reaches the pulp of the chickpeas, then it needs to break that down into a mush before it is small enough to enter the bloodstream. So, the whole chickpeas in the casserole will make the blood glucose rise much more slowly than when in the puréed hummus.

This is the case with most foods. For example, compare lentil and vegetable combo (*page 113*) to puréed lentil soup, or jacket potato to mashed potatoes, or seeded or grain bread to white sliced bread. For more examples, see the following table.

Choosing complex carbohydrate foods as meals and snacks will mean there's less room for fat, and if you're watching your weight, this can also help keep your calories down. Foods with a high glycaemic load are not bad foods. The key to healthy eating is getting the right mix of foods, which will not only ensure a better control of your blood glucose, but will also help you obtain the wide variety of nutrients needed for overall good health.

Glycaemic Load of Common Foods

Low GI Foods	Medium GI Foods	High GI Foods
Muesli	Rice	Cornflakes
Porridge	Potatoes	Bagels
Multi-grain bread	Rich Tea biscuits	French fries
Rye bread	Pitta bread	Glucose drinks
Pasta	White bread	Corn chips (Tortilla crisps)
Baked beans	Wholemeal bread	Crisped rice breakfast cereal
Lentils	Weetabix	Sports drinks
Apples	Shredded wheat	French baguette
Oranges	Couscous	Sugar-rich breakfast cereals
Yoghurt	Ice cream	

For precise quantities and a more extensive list, refer to *The Glucose Revolution* (*see Further Support and Information, page 195*).

Get Weight Wise

Any type of discipline that involves achieving something you value may require you to break through some kind of barrier. After all, chances are you've been eating the same way for years, so to change eating habits can be difficult – at least, if you perceive it to be so! If you interpret something as difficult or painful, your mind will wonder why on earth you would want this and reverts to what it interprets as pleasurable – like eating the doughnut and starting 'the diet' tomorrow! This inadvertently sabotages your goals in the process. By changing your thinking to interpret your goal as being pleasurable, enjoyable, fun and easy, you are far, far more likely to achieve what you set out to do. So, here's your chance to get creative with your waistline, so you can achieve long-term results.

The Fruit Salad Hypothesis

Hmm, doesn't sound too scientific, but this question is based on extensive research: are you an apple or a pear? Seriously, if your waist is bigger than your hips (an apple shape), you are more likely to suffer long-term conditions such as heart disease than if your waist is smaller than your hips (pear shaped). This is so significant that the British Dietetic Association Food First Campaign for 2002–2004, called *Weight Wise*, extensively published the following guidelines:

At risk waist measurement for European men: 94cm (37 inches)
At risk waist measurement for European and South Asian women: 80cm (32 inches)
At risk waist measurement for South Asian men: 90cm (36 inches)

Weighty Tips

- Have regular meals, preferably of a similar size each day. Keep to the amounts recommended by your dietitian or diabetes health-care professionals. If you miss meals, not only will this affect your blood glucose but undereating can also make you feel hungry and reach for less healthy foods.
- Remember to have five portions of fruit and vegetables each day. The health benefits are admirable, and when watching your weight these foods can help fill you up at a low-calorie cost.
- Plan meals ahead when possible. Have the right foods to hand, and less healthy foods out of sight.

- Use low-fat cooking methods: bake, grill (broil), roast without fat, microwave, steam, poach, chargrill, stir-fry and griddle (as in 'turkey koftas', *page 74*).
- If you have food cravings, it can help to know that they do pass. The longer you can resist the craving, the weaker it will become. But if you can't resist, don't fall into the trap of making yourself feel guilty. Instead, think how you might deal with a similar situation differently next time.
- Have to hand some vegetable or fruit nibbles such as carrots, melon and strawberries. Sugar-free jelly, a glass of tomato juice, chilled sugar-free drinks or a mug of low-calorie soup can be helpful when you feel like something extra.
- Enhance the natural flavours of your cooking with herbs, spices, garlic, chilli, lemon or lime juice, flavoured vinegars, tomato purée, a good flavoured stock, a splash of wine, soya sauce, hot pepper sauce, teryaki sauce, capers, a few olives and mustards.

Motivation

When you first decide to watch your weight, it's possible that your motivation is quite high. As time goes on, we all need a boost, so it's helpful to think about what getting fit and healthy means to you, not only in terms of how you look, but also the more important areas of your life.

Understanding what causes you to overindulge can be one of the most useful things you can do. When you come to terms with the underlying cause of this behaviour, you can begin to do something about it. There may be several interesting reasons that satisfy your need. These may include:

- comfort
- security
- boredom
- habit
- response to negative thoughts
- hunger
- when socializing
- to cope with stress or unpleasant feelings

Continuing to feed the habit, however, will only reinforce its effect. Looking for other, healthier ways to have this same need fulfilled will be of greater overall benefit.

To assess whether there are emotional needs that influence what and when you eat, you may like to keep a food and mood diary. Start by making a note of exactly what you eat over a few weekdays and a weekend. If you couple this with notes about how you were feeling at that particular time, you may start to see a connection between times when you feel like indulging and the mood you're in. This can better equip you to make lasting changes.

You can then explore filling your emotional needs with things other than food. Examples include taking up a hobby, exercising, studying or learning something new – anything that would bring you great enjoyment and help you develop (even more) fulfilling relationships. Think about it. What would have to happen for this need to be met in a healthy and functional way?

Think Well to be Well

The deeper motivational tips in this introduction are taken from a new concept in the management of diabetes, launched in 2002 by the Diabetes Research and Wellness Foundation in their publication *Think Well to be Well* (by Azmina Govindji and Nina Puddefoot).

Among another ideas, the concept focuses on your personal goals, based on the thinking that if you are crystal clear about *why* you would like to have a healthier lifestyle, you will increase your chances of having a strong and lasting motivation to succeed. You may want to ask yourself, for example, what having this new lifestyle or physique will do for you? How will having this new image affect other parts of your life – your confidence, your work performance, your social life, your belief in yourself? And how will it affect the way you interact with important people in your life – family, friends and colleagues? Once you truly know the impact and benefits the new lifestyle will have for you, the energy with which you move towards your goal will be vastly multiplied. And then you can apply this learning to other goals you want to achieve ... for more on this, visit www.thinkwelltobewell.com (*see Further Support and Information, page 195*).

Let's Get Physical

Physical activity helps your body release endorphins, natural painkillers, which can in turn help you combat stress and feel energized. You don't need to jog 10 times round the park or go to the gym every day in order to stay fit. Try to incorporate simple activities into your daily lifestyle and gradually work up to 30 minutes, five times a week. It's fine to have three ten-minute bursts of activity per day; you don't need to be exercising for 30 minutes at a time. Here are some ideas for getting active:

- Walk to the post box, take the dog out more often, take the kids for a brisk walk or simply park the car a bit further away. Try to walk at a pace that leaves you slightly out of breath.
- Use the stairs instead of the lift, or run up and down the steps at home a few times a day.
- Try skipping or jogging on the spot while watching your favourite television programme.
- Take up a sport you enjoy that fits into your routine. Swimming with the kids or line-dancing classes with a friend can be a fun way of working out.
- Remember that activity can be therapeutic, so tackling those garden weeds can have more benefits than you think.
- Yoga has a strong relaxing and calming effect.

Cheers!

If you have diabetes, there's no reason why you cannot enjoy a drink, unless of course you have been advised to avoid alcohol for another medical reason.

Observe the safe drinking limit for everyone: 21 to 28 units a week for men (or 3 to 4 units a day) and 14 to 21 units a week for women (or 2 to 3 units a day). These are maximum recommended amounts – it's better to drink less, and Diabetes UK recommends keeping to the lower recommended limits. Try to space your drinking throughout the week and to have two or three alcohol-free days each week.

Know Your Units

1 unit of alcohol = $1/2$ pint beer or lager = 1 pub measure of sherry, aperitif or liqueur = 1 standard glass of wine = 1 pub measure of spirits, e.g. vodka or gin

---

Safe Drinking

If you are taking insulin or certain tablets for your diabetes, alcohol can cause hypo-glycaemia (a 'hypo', or low blood glucose). Drinks that are higher in alcohol content, such as spirits, are more likely to cause a hypo. Here are a few guidelines which may help you prevent a hypo:

- Avoid drinking on an empty stomach. Always have something to eat with a drink (such as a handful of crisps or peanuts) and especially afterwards if you have been out drinking (such as biscuits, cereal or a sandwich). This is because the hypo-glycaemic effect of alcohol can last for several hours.
- Choose low-alcohol drinks in preference to those higher in alcohol. Avoid special diabetic beers or lagers, as these are higher in alcohol.
- If you enjoy spirits, try to use sugar-free/slimline mixers.
- If you count the amount of carbohydrate you eat, don't include the carbohydrate from alcoholic drinks.
- Try to alternate alcoholic and non-alcoholic drinks.
- If you are trying to lose weight, drink less alcohol (about a unit a day).

About the Recipes

These recipes will help you keep to a healthy diet without spending hours in the kitchen. The dishes have been created using convenient and healthier alternatives to standard ingredients, making them low in fat and sugar while being high in fibre. Meals are cooked in only a small amount of oil, and the oils chosen are unsaturat-ed, for the reasons outlined on page 6.

Each recipe has been carefully considered for its nutritional quality. Rest assured that the recipes are far lower in fat (particularly saturated fat) than traditional recipes, and that ingredients high in soluble fibre have been used wherever appropriate.

The serving suggestions are based on the nutritional value of each recipe, with ideas for boosting the carbohydrate content of the meal and vegetables to com-plement the dish. Although some dishes may already contain vegetables, it is a good idea to serve extra vegetables or salad.

When preparing meals, try to use only small amounts of salt. A high salt intake has been linked to high blood pressure. Choose good non-stick cookware so that you can cook in the minimum of oil without difficult washing-up!

Good luck!

Starters

This chapter contains quick and simple dishes to whet your appetite. Some of these first courses can also be served as light lunch or supper dishes, but should be accompanied by something starchy, such as a chunk of crusty bread, so that there is enough carbohydrate in your meal. The recipes range from hearty Lentil and Carrot Soup to a lighter Smoked Mackerel Pâté, and you are sure to find many healthy choices that become firm favourites.

The starters are designed to complement the main courses. Those based on vegetables, such as Baked Tomato and Olive Salad, are a good source of fibre and vitamins A (betacarotene) and C. Try to have two large portions of vegetables every day.

Tuna Cocktail

This salad makes an ideal starter served with bread.

Preparation time: 15 minutes
Serves: 4

- **1 tsp tomato purée (paste)**
- **1 tbsp reduced-calorie mayonnaise**
- **1 heaped tbsp low-fat fromage frais**
- **185g/6¹/₂ oz can tuna chunks in brine or spring water, drained**
- **¹/₂ green pepper, diced**
- **1 tbsp chopped fresh dill**
- **Black pepper**
- **4 tbsp finely shredded lettuce**
- **1 fresh lemon, sliced**

1 Mix the tomato purée (paste), mayonnaise and fromage frais in a bowl.
2 Add the tuna and green pepper. Season with the dill and pepper.
3 Divide the lettuce into four equal portions and place in the bottom of serving glasses.
4 Arrange the fish cocktail over the lettuce and chill. Just before serving, decorate with a slice of lemon.

Healthy Eating Notes

Use reduced-calorie mayonnaise instead of full-fat versions. Canned tuna in brine or water has half the calories of tuna in oil.

Tuna Lemon Pâté with Sweetcorn and Horseradish

The combination of lemon and horseradish gives this appetizer a delicious tang. Serve with either a coarse, grainy bread or wholemeal toast. If you don't want to get the food processor out, you could just mash the tuna with a fork for a rougher texture.

Preparation time: 15 minutes
Serves: 4

- **170g/6oz/1 cup canned, flaked tuna in brine or spring water (drained)**
- **55g/2oz/¹/₄ cup low-fat spread**
- **10ml/2 tsp horseradish sauce (or to taste)**
- **10ml/2 tsp lemon juice (or to taste)**
- **100g/3¹/₂ oz/¹/₂ cup canned sweetcorn kernels**
- **Wafer-thin slices of cucumber with skin left on (to garnish)**

1 Put the tuna and low-fat spread into a food processor or blender and whiz until smooth (or mash with a fork).
2 Add the horseradish and lemon juice to taste (if doing by hand, make sure they are well mixed in), and stir in the sweetcorn.
3 Spoon into ramekins and decorate, if liked, with thinly sliced cucumber.

Healthy Eating Notes

The sweetcorn adds taste and crunch as well as soluble fibre, valuable for good blood glucose levels.

Smoked Mackerel Pâté

A delicious starter with wholemeal bread or toast.

Preparation time: 15 minutes
Serves: 4

- **2 cooked smoked mackerel fillets (weighing about 115g/4oz each)**
- **140g/5oz low-fat fromage frais**
- **2 tbsp chopped chives**
- **1 tbsp lemon juice**
- **Pinch of cayenne pepper (optional)**

1 Remove the skin from the fish. Break the flesh into small pieces and mash with a fork. Be careful to remove any bones.
2 Mix together the fromage frais, chives, lemon juice and cayenne pepper (if using).
3 Blend the fish with this mixture using a fork. Serve chilled.

Healthy Eating Notes

The low-fat fromage frais makes a healthy alternative to cream cheese or double cream, which is often used in pâtés.

Fruity Chicken Liver Pâté

An unusual recipe, as the freshness of the grapes contrasts so well with the richness of the chicken livers. For convenience, use the small, thin-skinned, seedless variety of grapes. This pâté is delicious with French country bread, equally so on toast, and if you're making it for a dinner party, it actually improves with keeping in the fridge.

Preparation time: 5 minutes
Cooking time (including blending): 15 minutes
Serves: 4

- **30g/1oz/¹/₄ cup onion, finely chopped**
- **5ml/1 tsp sunflower oil**
- **115g/4oz/¹/₂ cup chicken livers, picked over for any gristle**
- **115g/4oz/¹/₂ cup low-fat soft cheese**
- **Salt and freshly ground black pepper to taste**
- **15ml/1 tbsp sherry or brandy (optional)**
- **55g/2oz/¹/₃ cup seedless white grapes, halved**

1 Sauté the onion gently in the oil for 2 or 3 minutes till soft.
2 Add the chicken livers and cook for a further 2 or 3 minutes till tender, but still pink on the inside.
3 Transfer to a blender or food processor along with the soft cheese and whiz until smooth.
4 Add seasoning to taste and, if you like, the sherry or brandy.
5 Mix in the grapes and spoon into four ramekins before serving.

Healthy Eating Notes

This is lower in fat than standard pâtés, and the grapes provide a good source of vitamin C.

Chilli Chicken Wings

I use ready-made crushed ginger and garlic from a jar for this recipe so that I spend less than 10 minutes on preparation. Just one bit of advice – serve with plenty of napkins!

Preparation and cooking time: 30 minutes
Serves: 4

- **12 skinless chicken wings**
- **1 tsp crushed ginger, from a jar**
- **2 tsp crushed garlic, from a jar**
- **1 tsp red chilli powder**
- **1 tbsp olive oil**
- **2 tsp honey**
- **2 tsp coarse-grain mustard**
- **1 tsp cider vinegar**
- **Salt and pepper**

1. Preheat the grill (broiler) to medium. Line a large flameproof dish with foil.
2. Put the chicken wings into a bowl. Add all the other ingredients and mix well.
3. Arrange the wings in the dish, making sure they don't overlap.
4. Cook under the grill for about 20 minutes, turning once or twice during cooking. Serve hot or cold.

Healthy Eating Notes

Remove the skin from all poultry before cooking to reduce the fat content. When you need to use fat in cooking, choose oil high in unsaturated fat, such as olive, rapeseed or sunflower oils.

Cocktail Kebabs with Yoghurt Dip

Each chunk of marinated chicken is threaded onto a cocktail stick and then dipped in a chilli-flavoured sauce. Although this is a starter, you can serve it as a main meal for two by stuffing the chicken kebabs into warmed (preferably wholemeal) pitta bread and smothering it with the dip and shredded lettuce. Yum!

Preparation time: 25 minutes
Cooking time: 10 minutes
Serves: 4

- **200g/7oz skinless chicken breasts, cut roughly into 2cm/1-inch cubes**

For the marinade
- **2 tsp olive oil**
- **1 tsp dried basil**
- **1 clove garlic, finely chopped or crushed**
- **2 tbsp light soy sauce**
- **Salt and pepper**

For the dip
- **2 x 150g/5fl oz pots low-fat natural yoghurt**
- **3 spring onions (scallions), green stems only, finely sliced**
- **Good pinch of red chilli powder**

1 Mix the marinade ingredients together.
2 Put the chicken pieces into a bowl and stir in the marinade. Set aside while you prepare the dip.
3 Preheat the grill (broiler) to high and line the grill pan with cooking foil. Mix the dip ingredients together and chill in the refrigerator.
4 Thread each chicken piece onto a cocktail stick and grill for about 10 minutes, turning once during cooking. Serve hot or cold with the yoghurt dip.

Healthy Eating Notes

Low-fat natural yoghurt makes an ideal base for a dip to accompany kebabs, chilli or curried dishes.

Summer Pea Soup with Bacon

This is simple to make, looks delicious and tastes even better! Frozen peas can be used and actually give a better colour than fresh, but avoid tinned peas as they just don't taste the same in this recipe. If time allows, serve chilled.

Preparation time: 5 minutes
Cooking time (including blending): 20 minutes
Serves: 4

- 1 small onion, finely chopped
- 570ml/20fl oz/2$^{1}/_{2}$ cups chicken stock
- 285g/10oz/2 cups fresh or frozen peas
- 285ml/10fl oz/1$^{1}/_{3}$ cups skimmed or semi-skimmed milk
- 45g/1$^{1}/_{2}$oz/$^{1}/_{4}$ cup smoked back bacon, diced
- Salt and white pepper to taste
- 45ml/1$^{1}/_{2}$fl oz/3 tbsp lower-fat Greek yoghurt (to garnish)
- A few freshly chopped chives (to garnish)

1 Simmer the onion in the chicken stock for about 5 minutes or until softened.
2 Add the peas and simmer for a further 5 minutes.
3 Add the milk and transfer to a blender or food processor. Whiz for a couple of minutes until smooth.
4 Strain or sieve the mixture back into the pan, add the bacon and cook for a further 3 or 4 minutes, then season to taste.
5 Serve each portion garnished with a swirl of Greek yoghurt and a scattering of freshly chopped chives

Healthy Eating Notes

Choosing lean bacon will help to keep the saturated fat content down.

Mediterranean Shrimp Soup

This is a 'second-helping soup' so make sure you have made plenty! Serve with crusty bread for a filling meal.

Preparation and cooking time: 30 minutes
Serves: 6

- 15ml/1 tbsp olive oil
- 285g/10oz/2^1/$_2$ cups onions, sliced
- 2 cloves garlic, crushed
- 340g/12oz/2^1/$_2$ cups aubergine (eggplant), peeled and diced
- 2 cans (each 395g/14oz/2 cups) chopped tomatoes
- 285ml/10fl oz /1^1/$_3$ cups dry white wine
- 2 tsp dried oregano
- 200g/7oz/1^1/$_2$ cups canned shrimps in brine, drained and rinsed
- 4 tbsp chopped parsley
- Juice of 1 lemon
- Freshly ground black pepper

1 In a large saucepan, heat the olive oil and add the onions and garlic.
2 Cover and let them sweat, but not colour, for 5 minutes until soft.
3 Add the diced aubergine (eggplant) and again cover for 5 minutes until soft.
4 Stir in the canned tomatoes, wine and oregano.
5 Cook for 15 minutes then add the shrimps, parsley and lemon juice.
6 Season with black pepper, heat through and serve.

Healthy Eating Notes

Shellfish contain cholesterol, but this is not harmful to your blood cholesterol. This is because blood cholesterol is more influenced by the amount of saturated fat you eat. Shrimps are low in saturated fat.

Herby Tomato Soup with Croutons

This is so simple you'll feel like you're cheating in the kitchen, and your friends need never know you haven't spent ages skinning, seeding, chopping and sieving the tomatoes. Passata (sieved tomatoes) can be bought in jars, bottles or cartons and should be a staple in any (cheating) cook's cupboard. The sugar in the recipe is essential – just a little, but enough to counteract the acidity in the tomatoes. For a vegetarian option, use vegetable rather than chicken stock.

Preparation time: 3 minutes
Cooking time: 10 minutes
Serves: 4

- **570ml/1 pint/2^1/$_2$ cups passata (sieved tomatoes)**
- **285ml/10fl oz/1^1/$_3$ cups chicken stock (from ^{1}/$_2$ cube)**
- **10ml/2 tsp red pesto**
- **5ml/1 tsp sugar**
- **Salt and freshly ground black pepper to taste**

For the croutons
2 x 45g/1^1/$_2$ oz slices white or wholemeal bread, crusts removed
45ml/1^1/$_2$fl oz/3 tbsp low-fat Greek yoghurt (to garnish)
4 small sprigs fresh basil (to garnish)

1 Put the passata and chicken stock into a pan and bring to the boil.
2 Add the pesto and sugar and season to taste.
3 Lower the heat and simmer for 5 minutes.
4 Meanwhile, toast the bread on both sides and dice into crouton shapes.
5 Serve each portion with a swirl of yoghurt and a sprig of fresh basil. Serve the croutons separately.

Healthy Eating Notes

Croutons are usually fried, but in this recipe they're toasted to keep the fat down. Low-fat yoghurt makes a healthier alternative to cream as a garnish.

Gazpacho

A chilled soup, perfect for a summer's day or a light starter. Cold soups are a pleasure to make because they are so simple and you can make them ahead of time.

Preparation time: 10 minutes
Serves: 6

- 1 litre/1³/₄ pints/4¹/₂ cups tomato juice, thoroughly chilled in the fridge
- Juice of 1 lemon
- 2.5ml/¹/₂ tsp white wine vinegar
- 2.5ml/¹/₂ tsp hot pepper sauce
- 370g/13oz/1¹/₂ cups low-fat natural Greek yoghurt
- ¹/₂ cucumber, peeled and diced
- 3 spring onions (scallions), finely chopped
- ¹/₂ tsp fresh dill, chopped
- Freshly ground black pepper

1 In a large bowl, mix the chilled tomato juice, lemon juice, vinegar, pepper sauce and yoghurt with a whisk until smooth and well blended.
2 Add the cucumber, spring onions (scallions) and dill, and season with black pepper.
3 Serve immediately and very cold. This can be stored in the fridge until needed.

Healthy Eating Notes

The low-fat Greek yoghurt is a healthier alternative to cream.

Leek and Potato Soup

No peeling or chopping of potatoes, no puréeing, just an instant mash potato mix with a fresh leek and you're well on your way! The mix is similar to potato flour, and you can use it to thicken the soup to your desired consistency. The crunchy leeks contrast beautifully with the smooth potato.

Accompany this with some crusty bread, or transform it into a main-meal soup by adding cooked peas or beans and sprinkling some reduced-fat Cheddar on top.

Preparation and cooking time: 15 minutes
Serves: 2

- **1 tbsp oil**
- **1 bay leaf**
- **2 fresh leeks, thinly sliced**
- **1 vegetable or chicken stock cube**
- **Pinch of tarragon**
- **30g/1oz instant mashed potato**
- **Salt and pepper**

1 Heat the oil and add the bay leaf.
2 Stir in the leeks and sauté for a couple of minutes to soften them.
3 Make the stock cube up to 285ml/$^1/_2$ pint/$1^1/_3$ cups with boiling water.
4 Add the stock and the tarragon to the leeks and bring back to the boil.
5 Remove the pan from the heat. Add the instant mashed potato and stir well to prevent any lumps from forming.
6 Season and serve.

Healthy Eating Notes

Although mashed potato is more quickly absorbed than whole potatoes, you can add pulses to the meal to promote good blood glucose control. If you do have more time, use fresh potatoes cut into small chunks. Serve when the potatoes are cooked but not mushy. Whole vegetables (rather than puréed) will not raise your blood glucose level so quickly. See the Introduction for more information on this.

Lentil and Carrot Soup

Vegetable soups make ideal starters or light meals. A large chunk of crusty bread is the perfect accompaniment.

Preparation time: 15 minutes
Cooking time: 20 minutes
Serves: 4

- **1 tsp corn oil**
- **15g/^{1}/$_2$ oz butter**
- **1 onion, chopped**
- **3 carrots, peeled and roughly chopped**
- **140g/5oz/^{3}/$_4$ cup red lentils**
- **^{1}/$_2$ tsp thyme or herbes de Provence**
- **1 litre/1^3/$_4$ pints/4^1/$_2$ cups vegetable stock**
- **Salt and pepper**

1 Heat a large pan with a lid. Add the oil and melt the butter in the oil over a low heat. Add the onion and sauté gently to soften.
2 Add the carrots and stir-fry for a few minutes.
3 Stir in the lentils, herbs and stock. Bring to the boil.
4 Cover and simmer for about 15–20 minutes, until the lentils are cooked. Season and serve.

Healthy Eating Notes

Carrots are a good source of betacarotene, which is converted by the body to vitamin A, an antioxidant vitamin.

Artichoke, Mushroom and Cherry Tomato Salad

This makes a very light and summery starter, ideal when followed by a poultry dish. You can add salad leaves if you like. Fine, lightly-cooked green beans are also nice tossed through it and, if you want something more substantial, baby new potatoes. Serve with crusty white or wholemeal bread to mop up the dressing.

Preparation time: 10 minutes
Serves: 4

- 340g/12oz/2$^1/_2$ cups canned artichoke hearts, drained
- 115g/4oz button mushrooms, wiped and halved
- 170g/6oz cherry tomatoes, left whole
- 60ml/4 tbsp oil-free French dressing
- 10ml/2 tsp extra-virgin olive oil
- A sprinkling of your favourite herb, chopped, such as chives, parsley, thyme, or a mixture (to garnish)

1 Combine the artichoke hearts, mushrooms and tomatoes in a bowl.
2 Mix the French dressing with the olive oil in a bottle or screw-top jar, shaking vigorously so that the two combine.
3 Pour over the salad and mix well.
4 Transfer to 4 individual plates or small bowls before serving, garnished with herbs.

Healthy Eating Notes

You'll cut down on the fat content dramatically if you don't include the olive oil in the dressing, but the taste will be very much sharper.

Lebanese Tabouleh Salad

Maybe it's a myth, but the story goes that if you eat this for lunch, the day can only get better. This salad is equally good as a supper starter or as a light snack. It's packed with flavour, very simple, and amazingly quick to prepare. Traditionally, it doesn't contain red and yellow peppers, but they look good and taste great! Do make sure you get fine bulgar wheat – the coarser type takes much longer to prepare.

Preparation time: 20 minutes
Serves: 4

- **200g/7oz/1 heaping cup fine bulgar wheat**
- **55g/2oz/$^1/_2$ cup spring onions (scallions), finely chopped**
- **115g/4oz/1 cup green (bell) pepper, diced**
- **115g/4oz/1 cup yellow (bell) pepper, diced**
- **170g/6oz cherry tomatoes, left whole**
- **30g/1oz/$^1/_2$ cup fresh parsley, finely chopped**
- **30ml/2 tbsp fresh coriander (cilantro), finely chopped**
- **45ml/3 tbsp lemon juice**
- **15ml/1 tbsp extra-virgin olive oil**
- **Salt and freshly ground black pepper**

1 Put the bulgar wheat into a large bowl, cover with boiling water and leave to soak for 15 minutes.
2 In the meantime, prepare the vegetables.
3 Transfer the bulgar wheat to a sieve, pressing down on it to remove any remaining liquid – it should be as dry as you can get it.
4 Turn into a serving bowl and mix with the spring onions (scallions), peppers, tomatoes and herbs.
5 Mix the lemon juice with the olive oil, season to taste and toss through the bulgar wheat mixture before serving. Serve chilled.

Healthy Eating Notes
The green and yellow peppers are a good source of vitamin C.

Baked Tomato and Olive Salad

A warming starter with a piquant flavour and lots of juices. Serve as a starter or light snack with plenty of French or ciabatta bread to mop up the juices.

Preparation time: 5 minutes
Cooking time: 10–15 minutes
Serves: 2

- **2 large tomatoes, sliced (around 140g/5oz each)**
- **10–12 pitted olives, halved**
- **3 spring onions (scallions), sliced**
- **1/2 tsp dried oregano**
- **Freshly ground black pepper**
- **1 tsp coarse-grain mustard**

1 Preheat the oven to 375°F/190°C/Gas Mark 5. Lightly grease or oil an ovenproof dish.
2 Mix all the ingredients together and place in the dish. Cover with foil and cook until the tomatoes have softened (about 10–15 minutes). Serve.

Healthy Eating Notes

Red, yellow and orange vegetables, such as tomatoes, yellow peppers and carrots, are rich in betacarotene. This is converted by the body to the antioxidant, vitamin A.

Olive Tapenade Bruschetta

Tapenade is an olive purée delicious with tomatoes or in a pasta dish. Available in jars from all supermarkets, it is a really useful addition to your store cupboard.

Bruschetta could also be topped with roasted peppers, artichokes, anchovies, capers or even olives themselves. A summer favourite that will transport you back to the shores of the Mediterranean.

Preparation time: 10 minutes
Serves: 4

- **15ml/1 tbsp olive oil**
- **2 cloves garlic, crushed**
- **370g/13oz/2 cups ripe tomatoes, sliced**
- **Freshly ground salt and black pepper**
- **4–5 sprigs basil, torn**
- **1 crusty loaf (approx 140g/5oz), cut into 8 slices**
- **10g/2 tsp tapenade**

1 Mix together the olive oil and crushed garlic and pour over the sliced tomatoes.
2 Season with salt and pepper and add in the torn basil leaves.
3 Grill the crusty slices of bread until golden, then spread with the tapenade.
4 Top with the flavoured tomato slices and serve immediately.

Healthy Eating Notes

The tomatoes in this recipe add lycopene, a valuable antioxidant.

Garlic Bread

Ready-made garlic paste, French bread and a hot grill (broiler) make this into a quick and easy aromatic starter, which goes especially well with pizzas and pasta dishes.

Preparation and cooking time: 10 minutes
Serves: 4

- **20cm/8-inch stick of French bread**
- **55g/2oz low-fat spread**
- **1 tsp garlic paste**
- **1/4 tsp mixed herbs**

1 Preheat the grill (broiler) to medium.
2 Cut the bread into 8 diagonal slices. Toast on one side.
3 Mix the spread, garlic and herbs together.
4 Spread the garlic mixture evenly over the untoasted side of the bread.
5 Grill the flavoured side till lightly browned.

Healthy Eating Notes

It's a good idea to serve extra bread with meals to boost the carbohydrate. The trouble is that it's usual to add some sort of spread. This recipe uses low-fat spread, which helps to keep the fat down. Remember that garlic bread bought in supermarkets or restaurants is likely to be made with lashings of butter – not the best of starters if you're trying to eat healthily!

Grilled Sardines with Fresh Orange

Fresh sardines are easy to cook and inexpensive. Choose large sardines such as the Cornish variety as they are not so fiddly with bones, and ask your fishmonger to clean them. Serve with crusty bread as a starter or boiled new potatoes and a tomato salad as a main course.

Preparation and cooking time: 20 minutes
Serves: 4

- **90ml/3fl oz /¹/₃ cup fresh unsweetened orange juice**
- **2 cloves garlic, crushed**
- **2 tbsp chopped parsley**
- **4 sardines (approx. 455g/1lb), heads removed and cleaned**
- **1 orange, peeled and segmented (to garnish)**

1 Mix together the orange juice, garlic and parsley in a dish.
2 Butterfly the sardines so they lie flat, by pressing down on the skin side.
3 Marinade the sardines in the juice mixture (flesh side downwards) for 5 minutes.
4 Preheat the grill (broiler) to high.
5 Place the sardines on a grill pan with some of the marinade mixture and grill for 4 minutes until ready.
6 Serve garnished with orange segments.

Healthy Eating Notes

Oily fish contains omega-3 fatty acids, which protect the body from heart disease. Try to eat oily fish once a week.

Nutty Prawns

The versatile and universal marinade works a treat with tiger prawns, tofu, chunks of meat – anything, in fact, that needs spicing up! You can use it immediately, such as on chicken wings, or you can marinade a whole roast in the fridge for up to 24 hours.

Preparation time: 5 minutes
Cooking time: 10 minutes
Serves: 4

- **285g/10oz/1^{1}/$_{2}$ cups tiger prawns, shelled and ready to cook**

For the marinade
- **2.5cm/1-inch piece root ginger, crushed**
- **2 cloves garlic, crushed**
- **15ml/1 tbsp groundnut (peanut) oil**
- **15ml/1 tbsp honey**
- **10ml/2 tsp coarse-grain mustard**
- **70g/2^{1}/$_{2}$ oz/4 tbsp smooth peanut butter**
- **30ml/2 tbsp light soy sauce**
- **15g/^{1}/$_{2}$ oz coriander (cilantro) leaves, finely chopped**
- **75ml/5 tbsp cold water**

1 Mix all the marinade ingredients together and brush over the prawns.
2 Stir-fry in a non-stick pan till cooked and still juicy. Add a little hot water if necessary and serve immediately.

Healthy Eating Notes

Peanut butter, be it smooth or crunchy, has a similar type of fibre to that found in dried fruit and beans, so it's helpful in diabetes as part of a healthy diet, although it is high in fat, so use in moderation. This marinade benefits from being cholesterol-free, and the peanut butter adds a range of vitamins including vitamin E and the B-vitamins.

Prawns with Apple and Cucumber

Preparation time: 10 minutes

Serves: 4

- 40g/1¹/₂oz reduced-calorie mayonnaise
- 40g/1¹/₂oz low-fat fromage frais
- 200g/7oz/2 cups frozen prawns, defrosted
- 1 apple, cubed
- 115g/4oz cucumber (around 7cm/3-inch stick), diced
- 1 tbsp raisins
- Pinch of cayenne pepper

1 Mix the mayonnaise and fromage frais together.
2 Add this dressing to all the other ingredients, except the cayenne pepper.
3 Divide the mixture into four individual serving dishes and sprinkle the cayenne pepper on top. Serve chilled, with bread rolls.

Healthy Eating Notes

Shellfish such as prawns contain cholesterol, but this is not harmful to your blood cholesterol. This is because blood cholesterol is more influenced by the amount of saturated fat you eat. Prawns are low in saturated fat.

Ham Cornets with Egg and Sweetcorn Mayonnaise

These little ham cornets make an excellent starter for a family evening meal, or can be served as a light lunch snack with crusty bread. If you want something more substantial, you can marry this with microwaved jacket potatoes. Substitute the sweetcorn for peas if you prefer.

Preparation time: 15 minutes
Cooking time: 10 minutes
Serves: 4

- **4 eggs**
- **115g/4oz/^{1}/$_2$ cup reduced-calorie mayonnaise**
- **100g/3^1/$_2$oz/^{1}/$_2$ cup canned sweetcorn kernels (drained weight)**
- **Salt and black pepper**
- **8 x 15g/^{1}/$_2$oz slices lean cooked ham**
- **8 small springs watercress (to garnish)**

1 Boil the eggs for 10 minutes then transfer to a colander and run under a cold tap to allow them to cool.
2 Remove the shells and place the boiled eggs in a bowl. Mash with the mayonnaise.
3 Stir in the sweetcorn and season lightly.
4 Form the ham into cone shapes, fill with the egg mixture and serve garnished with small springs of watercress.

Healthy Eating Notes

This recipe uses reduced-calorie mayonnaise to keep the fat content down.

Grilled Feta Cheese and Red Peppers

This is quite a high-fat starter, so ensure you choose a lower-fat main course. Or have this as a light meal with some warm crusty bread.

Preparation time: 5 minutes
Cooking time: 5 minutes
Serves: 2

- **115g/4oz feta cheese**
- **5ml/1 tsp ground cumin**
- **1 lettuce, torn**
- **15g/¹/₂oz fresh coriander (cilantro), torn**
- **1 red (bell) pepper, diced**
- **10ml/2 tbsp oil-free French dressing**
- **1 fresh orange**

1 Preheat the grill (broiler) and line a grill pan with foil. Cut the feta into eight thin slices and place on the foil.
2 Sprinkle on the ground cumin and grill, one side only, till the cheese starts to brown.
3 Lay the torn lettuce leaves and coriander (cilantro) on a plate with the red (bell) peppers and drizzle on the dressing.
4 Cut the orange in half and squeeze one half onto the dressed salad. Cut the other half into wedges.
5 Serve the feta cheese on top of the dressed salad leaves. Garnish with orange wedges.

Healthy Eating Notes

Red peppers are a valuable source of vitamin C and betacarotene.

Pork Satay with Peanut Sauce

Preparation and cooking time: 35 minutes

Serves: 4

- **225g/8oz lean pork, cut into bite-sized pieces**

For the marinade

- **1 tbsp light soy sauce**
- **1 tbsp Worcester sauce**
- **1/4 tsp Chinese five-spice powder**
- **1 clove garlic, crushed**
- **2 tsp sesame oil**
- **1 tsp honey**
- **Salt and pepper**

For the sauce

- **1 tbsp crunchy peanut butter**
- **1 tsp lemon juice**
- **2 tsp desiccated coconut**
- **1/4 tsp red chilli powder**

1 Preheat the grill (broiler) to a moderately high heat. Line the grill pan with foil.
2 Prepare the marinade by mixing all the ingredients together.
3 Put the pork into a bowl and coat with the marinade. Set aside.
4 Mix together all the ingredients for the sauce with 3 tbsp of cold water.
5 Thread the pork onto wooden skewers and grill (broil) until cooked, turning frequently.
6 Serve hot or cold with the peanut sauce.

Healthy Eating Notes

Lean pork can be just as low in fat as any other lean meat or poultry. Keep the fat down by using only small amounts of oil when cooking, as in this recipe.

Stuffed Mushrooms

Preparation and cooking time: 20 minutes
Serves: 4

- 8 large flat mushrooms (about 225g/8oz), stalks removed
- 30g/1oz Cheddar cheese, grated
- 1 tbsp chopped parsley
- 4 pitted olives, halved
- Freshly milled black pepper

1 Preheat the grill (broiler) to medium. Line the grill pan with foil.
2 Put the mushrooms into a frying pan (skillet). Add a little boiling water and cover with a lid. Cook the mushrooms for a couple of minutes only.
3 Drain the mushrooms and place them on the grill pan, rounded side down.
4 Mix the cheese with the parsley and use this to fill the mushrooms. Put half an olive in the centre of each mushroom and season to taste with the black pepper.
5 Grill (broil) for about a minute until the cheese has melted, and serve immediately.

Healthy Eating Notes

It's traditional to cook mushrooms in butter or oil, but you can simmer them in water without losing the flavour – and without the extra fat!

Florida Cocktail

Starters based on fruit and vegetables are much healthier than conventional starters such as pâtés and can help to balance a heavier main course. You can also serve this dish as a pudding – it contains fewer than 70 kilocalories a portion!

Preparation time: 10 minutes
Serves: 4

- **200g/7oz canned pineapple in natural juice, drained, reserving juice**
- **2 satsumas, peeled and segmented**
- **115g/4oz/²/₃ cup seedless grapes, halved**
- **2 kiwi fruits, peeled and sliced**

1 Mix the prepared fruits together with 90ml/3fl oz/¹/₃ cup of the reserved pineapple juice.
2 Divide the mixture into four individual serving glasses. Chill and serve.

Healthy Eating Notes

Fresh fruit is an excellent source of vitamin C and fibre. Try to eat three pieces of fruit a day.

Meat and poultry dishes

Everyone has different likes and dislikes when it comes to meat and poultry dishes. This chapter caters for all by including traditional British dishes, adapted so that they use healthier ingredients, interspersed with flavours from other parts of the world.

Most of these meals take a mere 20 minutes to prepare as they use shortcuts such as instant mashed potato and sauce mixes. Although more exotic dishes, such as Chicken with Cashew Nuts, are featured, there are no elaborate or time-consuming cooking methods. And you don't need to go to specialist shops for the ingredients.

It's a good idea to get into the habit of choosing lean meat and skinless poultry when shopping. Poultry in particular can make 'quick and easy' dishes. In some cases, you may find it more economical to buy poultry with the skin on – this can be easily removed during preparation. Cooking methods such as grilling (broiling) and stir-frying in the minimum amount of oil can help you reduce your fat intake even further. Choose unsaturated oils such as rapeseed, olive, corn and sunflower. Using non-stick cookware means you need less oil to prevent food from burning or sticking to the bottom of the pan. It also makes washing up easier!

You can make meat dishes healthier by adding beans and other pulses to recipes. This makes the meal go further and increases the amount of soluble fibre, which slows down the rise in blood glucose (sugar) after meals. This helps to keep your blood glucose within a healthy range, which is one of the key aims in the treatment of diabetes.

Meat-based dishes served as a main course are generally low in complex carbohydrates. Use the serving suggestions in this chapter to help you select appropriate accompaniments to create a balanced meal.

Lamb Steaks with Potato Ratatouille

You'll find that this particular mix of ratatouille marries well with chicken or turkey, but not duckling, as it's too rich. Use two large potatoes rather than, say, four small ones – saves time in the peeling!

Preparation time: 10 minutes
Cooking time: 25 minutes
Serves: 4

- 285g/10oz/2 cups raw potatoes, peeled and diced
- 15ml/1 tbsp olive oil
- 115g/4oz/1 cup onions, finely chopped
- 1 garlic clove, crushed
- 225g/8oz/2 cups courgette (zucchini), sliced
- 115g/4oz/1 cup baby aubergine (eggplant), diced
- 455g/1lb/2 cups chopped tomatoes (canned or fresh)
- 60ml/2fl oz/1/4 cup white wine
- 1 tsp caster sugar
- Good pinch dried herbes de Provence (Mediterranean mixed herbs)
- 4 x 115g/4oz lean lamb steaks, cut from the leg
- Salt and freshly ground black pepper to taste
- 4 small sprigs fresh rosemary (to garnish, optional)

1 Put the potatoes in a pan of salted water, bring to the boil and parboil for 5 minutes.
2 Meanwhile, heat the olive oil in a large, non-stick pan, and gently sauté the onion and garlic for 2–3 minutes until soft but not browned.
3 Add the rest of the vegetables, including the tomatoes, white wine, sugar and herbs, and bring to the boil.
4 When the potatoes are parboiled, drain them and tip into the pan along with the rest of the vegetables. Lower the heat and let the mixture simmer away happily, stirring occasionally.
5 Meanwhile, cook the lamb steaks under a medium grill (broiler) for 5–6 minutes each side, or until done as you like them.

6 Season the ratatouille to taste, and serve with the lamb steaks, garnished, if you like, with sprigs of fresh rosemary.

Healthy Eating Notes

The idea of combining ratatouille with potatoes makes sound sense for two reasons – the flavours go well together and the combination of fresh vegetables and potatoes makes for a hearty cocktail of nutrients.

Lamb Cutlets with Tomato and Mint Sauce

A refreshing and light sauce that combines well with the richness of lamb. This dish is ideal served with mashed potatoes to soak up the sauce and vegetables such as cauliflower, broccoli or green beans.

Preparation time: 5 minutes
Cooking time: 15 minutes
Serves: 4

- **4 lamb cutlets (approx. 100g/3^1/$_2$ oz each)**

For the sauce
- **680g/1^1/$_2$lb/3^1/$_2$ cups cherry tomatoes, halved**
- **10 leaves fresh mint (or 1 tsp mint sauce)**
- **1 tsp sugar**
- **Salt and freshly ground black pepper**

1 In a shallow, open pan, place the tomato halves with 30ml/2 tbsp of water and the mint leaves and simmer for 10 minutes until soft.
2 Add the sugar (and mint sauce if using) and then liquidize.
3 Season and reheat.
4 Meanwhile, grill (broil) the lamb cutlets under a medium heat until cooked (approx. 5 minutes), and serve with the sauce.

Healthy Eating Notes
When using red meat, choose lean pieces to keep the fat content down.

Spicy Lamb Burgers

These burgers are tastier than shop-bought varieties, with much less fat. Serve with a large helping of salad and a large bap, or if you're feeling really hungry some Southern Fries (*see page 148*).

Preparation time: 15 minutes
Cooking time: 15–20 minutes
Serves: 4

For the burgers
- **340g/12oz lean minced lamb**
- **1 onion, grated**
- **1 egg, beaten**
- **2 slices fresh wholemeal bread, made into breadcrumbs**
- **2 tsp curry powder**
- **1/4 tsp red chilli powder, or as desired**
- **1/4 tsp mustard**
- **Pinch of salt**

For serving
- **4 burger buns, warmed**
- **4 crisp lettuce leaves, washed and dried on paper towels**
- **3 tomatoes, sliced**

1 Preheat the grill (broiler) to medium. Mix together all the burger ingredients.
2 Divide the burger mixture into 4 portions and form into burger rounds a little larger than the buns.
3 Place directly onto the rack of the grill pan. Grill (broil) for about 15–20 minutes or until cooked thoroughly, turning the burgers halfway through cooking time.
4 Serve in warmed buns filled with the lettuce and tomatoes.

Healthy Eating Notes

Grilling (broiling) helps to drain off excess fat from the burgers as they cook.

Pan-fried Pork Scallopine with Lemon and Sage

These little escalopes are so quick and easy to do, and the tang of the lemon sauce contrasts beautifully with the richness of the pork. In Italy, they are traditionally made with veal, and they work equally well with escalopes of chicken or turkey.

Serve them with new or mashed potatoes or plain boiled rice. To enjoy them at their best, keep other side vegetables simple, such as fine green beans, spinach or broccoli.

Preparation time: 10 minutes
Cooking time: about 15 minutes
Serves: 4

- **4 x 115g/4oz lean escalopes of pork**
- **15ml/1 tbsp sunflower oil**
- **200ml/7fl oz/³/₄ cup pork or chicken stock (from ¹/₂ cube)**
- **60ml/2fl oz/¹/₄ cup dry white wine**
- **15ml/1tbsp lemon juice**
- **4 small sprigs fresh sage**
- **4 tsp cornflour (cornstarch)**
- **¹/₂ tsp caster (confectioner's) sugar (or to taste)**
- **Salt and white pepper to taste**
- **8 wafer-thin slices lemon (to garnish)**

1 Beat the escalopes with a rolling pin or mallet (or even a milk bottle) until very, very thin.
2 Heat the oil in a large, non-stick frying pan (skillet) and sauté the escalopes for 3 minutes on each side (you may have to do them in 2 batches). Remove from the pan with a slotted spoon and keep warm.
3 Add the stock, wine, lemon juice and sprigs of sage to the pan and bring to the boil.

4 Mix the cornflour (cornstarch) to a paste with a little water, stir into the pan and continue stirring until the sauce thickens. Cook for a further minute then season, add the caster (confectioner's) sugar and heat until dissolved.

5 Serve the escalopes with the sauce poured over and garnished with wafer-thin slices of lemon.

Healthy Eating Notes

Choosing lean escalopes of pork helps keep the fat content down.

Pork with Fresh Plums

Plums make a great low-fat base for a delicious pink sauce with a slightly Oriental taste.

Preparation time: 5 minutes
Cooking time: 25 minutes
Serves: 4

- 500g/18oz/3 cups fresh plums, halved
- 285ml/10fl oz/1¹/₃ cups chicken stock
- 10ml/2 tsp sunflower oil
- 1 large onion (225g/8oz/2 cups), finely sliced
- 170g/6oz/3 cups white cabbage, finely shredded
- 395g/14oz/2 cups lean pork fillet, cut into bite-sized pieces
- Freshly ground black pepper

1 Simmer the plums in chicken stock for 5 minutes.
2 Remove the stones and skins and purée the flesh and stock.
3 In a large frying pan (skillet), heat the oil and cook the onion until soft.
4 Add the raw, shredded cabbage and continue to cook for a further 3 minutes.
5 Add the pork pieces to brown and then the puréed plums.
6 Season and simmer for 15 minutes before serving.

Healthy Eating Notes

Serve with basmati rice, which has a low glycaemic index (see *Introduction*).

Pork Steaks with Creamy Mustard Sauce

The pork steaks are enhanced by the taste of mustard to make a delicious and convenient dish.

Preparation time: 5 minutes
Cooking time: 15 minutes
Serves: 4

- **10ml/2 tsp sunflower oil**
- **4 lean pork steaks (approx. 115g/4oz each), trimmed of any fat**
- **1 onion (approx. 85g/3oz/²/₃ cup), finely chopped**
- **140ml/5fl oz/²/₃ cup hot chicken stock**
- **170g/6oz/²/₃ cup low-fat natural yoghurt**
- **4 tsp wholegrain mustard**

1 Heat a heavy-based frying pan (skillet) or griddle. Add the oil and pan-fry the pork steaks for 10 minutes, turning occasionally until cooked through.
2 Remove from the pan and keep hot, ready for serving.
3 Add the onion to the residues in the frying pan, and cook until soft.
4 Add the hot stock and cook for another 5 minutes.
5 Remove from the heat and stir in the yoghurt and mustard.
6 Gently reheat, stirring continuously, and serve poured over the pork steaks.

Healthy Eating Notes

Pork steaks are now much leaner and consequently lower in fat, and the yoghurt makes an excellent low fat substitute for cream.

Pork Burgers

Pork burgers are great served on a grilled bun piled high with lettuce and relish – much better than any shop-bought burger.

Preparation and cooking time: 25 minutes
Serves: 4

- **1 dessert apple (approx. 85g/3oz/^{3}/$_4$ cup)**
- **455g/16oz/2 cups lean, finely minced pork**
- **15g/^{1}/$_2$ oz chives, chopped**
- **30g/1oz/^{1}/$_4$ cup wholemeal breadcrumbs**
- **Salt and freshly ground black pepper**

1 Preheat the grill (broiler) to medium-high.
2 Peel and then grate the apple.
3 Put the grated apple in a large bowl with all the other ingredients.
4 Mix thoroughly by hand to ensure it is completely mixed.
5 Divide the mixture into 4 and press each into a burger shape.
6 Place on a wire rack in the grill and cook for 15 minutes, turning once, until there is no trace of pink in the centre.

Healthy Eating Notes

The recipe calls for lean pork and the burgers are cooked under the grill (broiler) to help keep the fat down.

Sweet and Sour Pork

Serve with plenty of boiled rice or noodles.

Preparation and cooking time: 20 minutes
Serves: 4

- **340g/12oz lean pork tenderloin fillet, cut into 1cm/$^1/_2$-inch cubes**
- **1 tbsp cornflour (cornstarch)**
- **1 tbsp corn oil**
- **1 tbsp light soy sauce**
- **1 green (bell) pepper, cut into strips**

For the sauce

- **1 tbsp cornflour (cornstarch)**
- **2 tsp caster (confectioner's) sugar**
- **1 tbsp white wine vinegar**
- **2 tbsp fresh orange juice**
- **1 tbsp light soy sauce**
- **2 tsp tomato purée (paste)**

1 Coat the pork in the cornflour (cornstarch). Heat the oil in a non-stick pan. Fry the pork cubes over a high heat for about 5 minutes until brown. Add a little hot water if they begin to burn.
2 Stir in the soy sauce and green peppers and cook for a few minutes.
3 Mix the sauce ingredients together with 3 tbsp of water. Add the sauce to the pan and stir until it thickens. Add a little hot water if you prefer the sauce to be less thick.

Healthy Eating Notes

Sweet and sour dishes can be high in fat and sugar. This is because the pork is often fried in batter and a lot of sugar is used in the sauce. In this recipe, instead of batter, the pork is stir-fried in a little oil and its own juices.

Liver and Bacon Kebabs

This is a variation of the traditional dish. Instead of serving with mashed potatoes, try it with plain boiled rice and drizzled with balsamic vinegar.

If using wooden skewers, remember to soak them in water for 10 minutes before use to prevent them burning.

Preparation time: 15 minutes

Cooking time: 10 minutes

Serves: 4

- 285g/10oz/1¼ cups liver (chicken or lamb is recommended), soaked in milk
- 4 cup lean back smoked bacon rashers
- 115g/4oz/¾ cup cherry tomatoes
- 170g/6oz/1½ cups courgette (zucchini), sliced thinly
- 1 onion (approx. 85g/3oz/⅔ cup), peeled, cut into quarters then divided again
- 115g/4oz/1 cup button mushrooms, washed
- 5ml/1 tsp olive oil

1 Soak the liver in milk for 5 minutes to remove any bitterness.
2 Meanwhile, stretch the bacon rashers with the back of a knife and cut each into two lengthways. Roll each piece up into a small roll.
3 Preheat the grill (broiler) to high.
4 Drain the milk from the liver and cut into bite-sized pieces.
5 Thread the liver pieces, cherry tomatoes, courgette slices, onion pieces, mushrooms and bacon rolls onto 4 skewers and place on a large grill pan.
6 Brush with the olive oil and grill under a high heat for 10 minutes.

Healthy Eating Notes

Liver is an excellent source of iron, protein and B-vitamins, including B12.

Broccoli and Ham Pasta Spirals

A quick and easy pasta dish that looks especially good if made with three-coloured pasta spirals. If you want a stronger flavour, you can substitute large, sliced mushrooms for the button mushrooms. And remember, the most important preparation tip is to cook the pasta al dente, so it still has a bite and does not become very soft.

Preparation time: 5 minutes
Cooking time: 15–20 minutes
Serves: 4

- 300g/10^1/$_2$ oz/3^1/$_2$ cups pasta spirals
- 100g /3^1/$_2$ oz/^{1}/$_2$ cup passata
- 125g/4^1/$_2$ oz/1^1/$_2$ cups button mushrooms
- 140g/5oz/^{2}/$_3$ cup lean smoked ham pieces
- 2 tbsp pesto
- 2 tsp tomato purée (paste)
- 300g/10^1/$_2$ oz/3^1/$_2$ cups broccoli florets, cooked but still crunchy
- Freshly ground black pepper
- Basil leaves (to garnish)

1 Cook the pasta spirals according to the instructions on the packet, then drain.
2 Heat the passata in a large pan and add the button mushrooms, cooking for 3 minutes.
3 Add the ham pieces, pesto and tomato purée, and mix well.
4 Stir in the broccoli florets and cooked pasta spirals and cook until thoroughly heated.
5 Season with freshly ground black pepper and serve decorated with fresh basil leaves.

Healthy Eating Notes

Pasta is nutritious and filling, with a low glycaemic index (*see Introduction*).

Tagliatelle with Ham and Cream

A rich-tasting Italian dish made with fresh basil and garlic. Serve with a large salad in fat-free dressing, and try not to have a high-fat starter.

Preparation and cooking time: 20 minutes
Serves 3

- **225g/8oz tagliatelle**
- **2 tsp oil**
- **1 onion, finely sliced**
- **2 cloves garlic, crushed**
- **225g/8oz mushrooms, sliced**
- **90ml/3fl oz/¹/₃ cup half-fat single (coffee) cream**
- **115g/4oz cooked ham, chopped**
- **15g/¹/₂ oz packet fresh basil leaves, chopped**
- **Salt and pepper**

1 Cook the pasta according to the instructions on the packet.
2 Heat the oil in a large non-stick pan over a medium heat. Add the onion and garlic and cook for a couple of minutes to soften.
3 Add the mushrooms and stir-fry for a few minutes until just cooked.
4 Pour in the cream. Add the drained pasta, ham, basil and seasoning and stir well. Heat through and serve.

Healthy Eating Notes

Pasta dishes are filling and nutritious, and although this is a rich dish, it uses half-fat cream as opposed to standard full-fat versions.

Peppery Beef Strips on Giant Croutons

A classy recipe that is wonderful served at a special meal accompanied by a variety of lightly cooked vegetables. The pepper sauce is not hot, but do watch out when you bite down on the peppercorns!

Serving the meat and sauce on top of a large, crunchy crouton gives a great texture and makes sure that you do not waste any of the delicious sauce.

Preparation time: 5 minutes
Cooking time: 20 minutes
Serves: 4

- **8 small rounds of bread, cut from a French stick (approx. 230g/8oz in total)**
- **5ml/1 tsp olive oil**
- **5ml/1 tsp sunflower oil**
- **1 onion (approx. 85g/3oz/^{2}/$_3$ cup), finely sliced**
- **340g/12oz/1^1/$_2$ cups lean sirloin steak, trimmed and cut into strips**
- **285ml/^{1}/$_2$ pint/1^1/$_3$ cups hot beef stock**
- **4 tsp (pink) peppercorns in brine, drained**
- **170g/6oz/^{2}/$_3$ cup low-fat natural yoghurt**
- **Chopped parsley (to garnish)**

1 Preheat the oven to high (220°C/425°F/Gas Mark 7).
2 Place the bread rounds on an ovenproof tray and brush on both sides with the olive oil.
3 Cook in the oven for 10 minutes until crispy.
4 In a heavy-based frying pan (skillet), heat the sunflower oil and cook the sliced onion until soft.
5 Add the beef strips and cook for 3 minutes.
6 Remove the onion and beef from the pan and keep hot.
7 Add the stock and the peppercorns to the frying pan.
8 Simmer for 5 minutes then add the yoghurt plus the beef and onion mixture.

9 Heat thoroughly, stirring continuously.

10 To serve, place the large bread croutons on plates and pile the beef strips in pepper sauce on top.

11 Garnish with chopped parsley.

Healthy Eating Notes

The croutons add filling carbohydrate, so all you need are some lightly cooked vegetables to make this into a complete meal.

Meatloaf

Cooking these individually means that the dish can be prepared quickly. However, it is just as tasty cooked in a small loaf tin for 50–60 minutes and sliced. Serve hot or cold with potatoes and salad. Any leftover meatloaf makes a perfect sandwich filling.

Preparation and cooking time: 30 minutes
Serves: 4

- **395g/14oz/1³/₄ cups lean minced beef**
- **55g/2oz/¹/₂ cup onion, finely diced**
- **55g/2oz/²/₃ cup mushrooms, finely diced**
- **2 tbsp chopped fresh herbs (e.g. chives and parsley)**
- **1 egg white**
- **Pinch of salt and freshly ground black pepper**

1 Preheat the oven to 190°C/375°F/Gas Mark 5.
2 In a large bowl, mix together all the ingredients well with your hands.
3 Divide the mixture into 4 and press into the hollows of an indented baking tray (a large Yorkshire pudding tray or individual tartlet tray with hollows about 8cm/3 inches in diameter and 1cm/¹/₂-inch deep is good).
4 Cover with foil and bake for 20–25 minutes until cooked.

Healthy Eating Notes

Using lean minced beef helps keep the fat content down.

Beef Curry

When you think about preparing a curry, you imagine that you'll be slaving over a hot stove for hours. This quick and easy method needs only one pan and a bit of stirring. Otherwise, just leave it to cook on its own while the flavours develop and the aroma just manages to escape from a tightly closed lid. Complement this dish with some plain boiled rice, a large portion of mixed salad and some Cucumber and Mint Raita (*see page 167*).

Preparation time: 10 minutes
Cooking time: 20 minutes
Serves: 4

- **1 tbsp corn oil**
- **1 tsp crushed ginger, from a jar**
- **1 tsp crushed garlic, from a jar**
- **2 fresh green chillies, chopped**
- **1 tsp turmeric**
- **1 heaped tsp curry powder**
- **455g/1lb rump steak, cut into bite-size pieces**
- **115g/4oz canned chopped tomatoes**
- **2 tsp tomato purée (paste)**
- **115ml/4fl oz/^{1}/$_2$ cup hot water**
- **Salt**
- **15g/^{1}/$_2$oz packet fresh coriander (cilantro), chopped**

1 Heat a large non-stick saucepan with a lid. Add all the ingredients except the coriander (cilantro) one at a time, stirring after every few additions.

2 Cover and cook over a medium heat for about 20 minutes, stirring occasionally until the steak is tender.

3 Stir in the coriander (cilantro), heat through and serve.

Healthy Eating Notes

Choose lean beef wherever possible. This will help you to limit the amount of saturated fat you eat. To make this dish go further, add 340g/12oz of peas 10 minutes before the end of cooking time.

Warm Chicken Salad

An impressive main-course salad that would also serve 6 as a starter. Using coloured salad leaves and cherry tomatoes makes it look attractive. It is so simple to prepare – even the salad dressing can be made in advance and kept in the fridge until needed.

Cooked noodles could be included at stage 4 or the salad could be served with boiled new potatoes on the side.

Preparation time: 5 minutes
Cooking time: 10 minutes
Serves: 4

- **395g/14oz/1¹/₂ cups chicken breast fillets, cut into bite-sized pieces**
- **1 tbsp plain (all purpose) flour**
- **115g/4oz/1 cup mangetout**
- **15ml/1 tbsp sunflower oil**
- **140g/5oz/1 cup cherry tomatoes, halved**
- **85g/3oz/1 cup mixed salad leaves**
- **30g/1oz/¹/₄ cup spring onions (scallions), chopped**
- **1 tsp chives, chopped finely (to garnish)**
- **Large pinch sesame seeds (to garnish)**

For the dressing
- **15ml/1 tbsp balsamic vinegar**
- **15ml/1 tbsp sesame seed oil**
- **15ml/1 tbsp soy sauce**

1 Roll the chicken pieces in the flour to coat them.
2 Cook the mangetout in boiling water for 2 minutes then drain.
3 Make the dressing by mixing all the ingredients together.
4 Heat the sunflower oil and cook the chicken pieces for 5 minutes, turning once. Add the mangetout and cherry tomatoes and cook for a further 2 minutes.
5 Arrange the salad leaves and chopped spring onions on the serving plates.

6 Pile the warm chicken and vegetable mixture on top of the salad and drizzle over the dressing.

7 Sprinkle with the chives and sesame seeds before serving.

Healthy Eating Notes

The colourful mangetout and tomatoes provide valuable antioxidant vitamins.

Chicken with Red Pepper Sauce

This could also be made with yellow peppers – a ribbon of each could be spooned over the chicken to give contrasting colours.

By adding extra yoghurt to the sauce to thin it down you can make a chilled soup!

Preparation time: 10 minutes
Serves: 4

- **2 red (bell) peppers (approx. 170g/6oz each)**
- **1 clove garlic, chopped**
- **15ml/3 tsp dry sherry**
- **425g/15oz/2 cups low-fat natural yoghurt**

Serve with
- **4 cooked chicken breasts (approx. 115g/4oz each)**
- **Watercress (to garnish)**

1 Remove the skins from the red peppers by blackening the peppers over a flame and then scraping the skin off.
2 Remove the stalks and take out the seeds.
3 Chop the peppers finely and place in a blender with the chopped garlic and the sherry.
4 Blend until smooth and then mix in the yoghurt.
5 Serve chilled with cold grilled chicken and garnish with watercress.

Healthy Eating Notes

An alternative to creamy sauces or mayonnaise, red pepper sauce is delightfully light and low in calories.

Smoked Chicken with Pasta Shells

A simple and refreshingly light pasta dish with a unique combination of flavours. Wonderful served with fresh rocket leaves on top.

Preparation and cooking time: 15 minutes
Serves: 4

- **285g/10oz/3$^{1}/_{3}$ cups pasta shells**
- **15ml/1 tbsp olive oil**
- **200g/7oz/1$^{1}/_{4}$ cups cooked, smoked chicken, diced**
- **425g/15oz/2$^{1}/_{2}$ cups tomatoes, diced**

1 Cook the pasta according to the instructions on the packet.
2 Drain and return to the pan. Turn off the heat.
3 Add the smoked chicken pieces and mix well.
4 Immediately before serving, add the tomato dice and mix through quickly.

Healthy Eating Notes

Pasta is nutritious and filling, with a low glycaemic index (*see Introduction*).

Chicken Pulau

A one-pot Asian dish that is wonderfully spicy and aromatic. It contains chicken, rice and vegetables and is substantial enough for any appetite. For convenience, I usually use crushed ginger and garlic from a jar. If you prefer a less hot and spicy dish, remove the seeds from the green chillies during preparation.

All you need to serve with this to make a tasty low-fat meal is some fresh mixed salad and low-fat natural yoghurt.

Preparation time: 15 minutes
Cooking time: 20 minutes
Serves: 4

- **2 tbsp corn oil**
- **1 onion, finely chopped**
- **3 tsp cumin seeds**
- **1 tsp crushed ginger**
- **1 tsp crushed garlic**
- **2 green chillies, finely chopped**
- **285g/10oz skinless chicken breasts, chopped into bite-size pieces**
- **140g/5oz low-fat natural yoghurt**
- **5 tbsp sieved tomatoes**
- **285g/10oz frozen mixed vegetables**
- **Salt**
- **500ml/18fl oz/2¼ cups boiling water**
- **225g/8oz/1 heaping cup basmati or long-grain rice**

1 Heat the oil in a large saucepan with a lid.
2 Add the onion, cumin seeds, ginger, garlic and chillies. Fry gently over a medium heat for a couple of minutes.
3 Increase the heat and add the chicken. Brown for about 3–5 minutes.
4 Stir in the yoghurt, tomatoes, vegetables and salt. Simmer for a couple of minutes.
5 Add the boiling water and bring back to the boil.

6 Stir in the rice, cover and cook over a medium heat until the water is absorbed (about 20 minutes). Serve.

Healthy Eating Notes

The combination of rice, vegetables and lean meat in this recipe provides a good mix of starchy carbohydrate, fibre and vitamins while keeping an eye on the fat content.

Honeyed Drumsticks

Balance this dish by serving with some starchy carbohydrate, such as boiled new potatoes in their skins. Accompany these with a couple of servings of colourful vegetables, such as French beans and sweetcorn. Alternatively, this makes a great outdoor dish if served with some crusty bread and mixed salads.

Preparation time: 5 minutes
Cooking time: 30 minutes
Serves: 4

- **2 skinless chicken drumsticks**
- **2 tsp honey**
- **2 tsp sesame oil**
- **1 tbsp soy sauce**
- **1 tbsp Worcester sauce**
- **Coarsely ground black pepper**

1 Preheat the grill (broiler) to medium.
2 Line the grill pan with cooking foil and put the drumsticks into the dish.
3 Mix all the other ingredients together and coat the chicken.
4 Grill (broil), turning frequently, for about 30 minutes or until the chicken is cooked and the juices run clear when the chicken is pierced with a fork.

Healthy Eating Notes

Removing the skin from chicken significantly reduces the fat content. Using a small amount of honey, as in this recipe, will not be harmful to your blood glucose level.

Lemony Roast Chicken

Chicken breasts are sealed in foil with fresh lemon slices, whole cloves of garlic and fresh basil leaves. Let the flavours develop in the oven while you prepare the accompaniments. To serve, add some Sesame Green Beans (*see page 161*) with a starchy carbohydrate such as Vegetable Rice (*see page 129*) or boiled new potatoes in their skins.

Preparation time: 5 minutes
Cooking time: 25–30 minutes
Serves: 4

- **4 skinless chicken breasts (about 455g/1lb total weight)**
- **4 cloves garlic, peeled only**
- **15g/¹/₂oz packet fresh basil leaves**
- **2 fresh lemons, sliced**
- **Salt and pepper**
- **2 tsp olive or rapeseed oil**

1 Preheat the oven to 375°F/190°C/Gas Mark 5. Cut pieces of foil large enough to wrap each chicken breast.
2 Place each chicken breast with one whole clove of garlic, a quarter of the basil, a few slices of lemon and seasoning onto a piece of foil.
3 Drizzle each 'parcel' with a little oil. Loosely wrap the chicken pieces and roast until cooked.

Healthy Eating Notes

Using fresh herbs and garlic to season dishes enables you to cut down on the amount of salt needed in cooking. Eating too much salt is associated with a greater risk of high blood pressure.

Chicken with Cashew Nuts

A familiar Chinese favourite cooked with traditional ingredients. To save time, I use a frozen pack of Chinese vegetables, which contains mangetout and baby sweetcorn. Choose whichever vegetables you prefer, fresh or frozen. To serve, some plain boiled rice or noodles are all you need.

Preparation and cooking time: 20 minutes
Serves: 4

For the chicken
- **1 tbsp plain flour**
- **Black pepper**
- **2 tbsp light soy sauce**
- **2 skinless chicken breasts (weighing about 340g/12oz in total), cut into bite-sized pieces**
- **2 tsp corn or groundnut (peanut) oil**
- **30g/1oz cashew nuts**

For the vegetables
- **1 tsp sesame oil**
- **6 spring onions (scallions), cut into thick, diagonal slices**
- **1 clove garlic, crushed**
- **1cm/^{1}/$_2$-inch root ginger, chopped or crushed (optional)**
- **455g/1lb frozen or fresh Chinese mixed vegetables**
- **2 tbsp light soy sauce**
- **^{1}/$_2$ tsp Chinese five-spice powder or pinch black pepper**

1 Season the flour with the pepper. Stir the soy sauce into the chicken and then coat the chicken in the seasoned flour.
2 Heat a wok or wide-based non-stick pan and add the oil. Stir-fry the chicken over a high heat until well browned (about 5–6 minutes).
3 Add the cashew nuts and continue to stir-fry for a couple of minutes. Remove the chicken and cashew nut mixture, set aside and keep warm.
4 Heat the sesame oil in the same pan or wok. Add the onions, garlic and ginger (if using) and stir-fry for a few minutes.

5 Add the vegetables, soy sauce and five-spice powder (or pepper). Stir-fry for about 5 minutes.

6 Return the chicken mixture to the pan and heat through for a few minutes to let the flavours mix well.

Healthy Eating Notes

Quick cooking, such as stir-frying, is an excellent way to preserve nutrients and cut down on fat. Soy sauce contains a lot of salt, so there's no need to add more. Always serve stir-fried dishes with plenty of boiled rice or noodles so that you fill up on starchy carbohydrates.

Chicken Liver and Fennel

Chicken livers have a delicate taste compared to other offal. Make sure you don't overcook the liver as it can then become tough. The fennel used in this recipe has a mild aniseed flavour. This recipe makes a good alternative to the standard 'liver and onions' dish. If you like sweet and sour flavours, pour in a few tablespoons of fresh orange juice just before serving. Try serving with Sesame Green Beans (see page 161) and boiled new potatoes in their skins.

Preparation and cooking time: 30 minutes
Serves: 2

- **2 tsp corn oil**
- **225g/8oz fennel, halved and thinly sliced**
- **Salt and pepper**
- **1 tbsp plain flour**
- **225g/8oz chicken livers**
- **3 tbsp chopped parsley**
- **1 tbsp red wine vinegar**

1 Heat the oil over a moderately high heat. Stir-fry the fennel for about 3 minutes.
2 Add the salt and pepper to the flour. Use this seasoned flour to coat the liver.
3 Add the liver to the pan and cook very quickly for about 5–10 minutes, stirring gently from time to time.
4 Slowly mix in the parsley and remove from the heat. Pour in the vinegar. This should make a sizzling sound – serve immediately.

Healthy Eating Notes

Liver is an excellent source of iron, protein and B-vitamins, including B12. Drinking some unsweetened orange juice with it will help you to make more use of the iron in the liver, as the vitamin C from the juice helps your body to absorb the iron more efficiently. Serve this dish with vegetables and a starchy carbohydrate.

Turkey Koftas

These sausage-like kebabs can be served in a variety of ways. Try them with saffron rice and grilled vegetables. Alternatively, fill some warm pitta bread with salad, place the turkey koftas on top and add some natural yoghurt for a plate-free meal.

Preparation time: 10 minutes
Cooking time: 15 minutes
Serves: 4

- 340g/12oz/1½ cups lean turkey breast, minced
- 30g/1oz/⅔ cup fresh chopped herbs (oregano, chives and parsley are a good combination)
- 2 cloves garlic, crushed
- Juice of ½ lemon
- Salt and freshly ground black pepper
- 5ml/1 tsp olive oil

1 Preheat the grill (broiler) to medium.
2 In a large bowl, combine all the ingredients except the oil and mix well with your hands.
3 Divide the mixture into 4 and roll into sausages, approximately 2cm/¾ inch in diameter.
4 Guide a metal skewer through the kofta and place on a grill pan.
5 Brush with olive oil and grill until cooked (approx. 15 minutes).

Healthy Eating Notes

Turkey breast is very low in fat and makes an excellent alternative to fattier meats.

Turkey Fricassee

A fricassee is a white stew of poultry and vegetables, first fried in butter and then cooked in stock with the addition of cream and egg yolks. This recipe is adapted to keep the saturated fat down by using Greek yoghurt and chicken stock to make an appetizing sauce for turkey, carrots and green peppers. Buy fresh turkey breasts from the supermarket or make this into a great Boxing Day treat using leftovers. Add a dash of white wine for that special occasion. Serve with boiled rice.

Preparation and cooking time: 30–35 minutes
Serves: 4

- **1 tbsp plain flour**
- **Salt and pepper**
- **4 skinless turkey breasts (weighing around 170g/6oz each), cut into bite-size chunks**
- **2 tsp corn or rapeseed oil**
- **1 onion, finely chopped**
- **2 cloves garlic, crushed**
- **1 chicken stock cube**
- **3 carrots, diced**
- **1 green (bell) pepper, diced**
- **115g/4oz Greek yoghurt**
- **4 tbsp fresh parsley, chopped**

1 Mix the flour with the seasoning and use this to coat the turkey pieces.
2 Heat the oil in a non-stick pan. Add the onion and garlic and fry for a few minutes to soften.
3 Make the chicken stock cube up to 250ml/9fl oz/1¼ cups with hot water.
4 Add the turkey to the pan and brown over a medium heat for about 5 minutes, adding a little of the stock if it sticks to the bottom.
5 Stir in the carrots and remaining stock. Cover and simmer for 5 minutes.
6 Add the peppers and allow to cook, covered, for a further 5 minutes.

7 Stir in the yoghurt and parsley. Warm through and adjust the seasoning if necessary.

Healthy Eating Notes

Greek yoghurt contains more fat than most other yoghurts. However, it is substantially lower in fat than cream yet still has a rich, creamy flavour.

Pan-fried Turkey Breasts

Turkey is available all year round and is often cheaper outside the Christmas season. The turkey in this recipe has a wonderful charred appearance. You can serve with traditional roast potatoes and Brussels sprouts, or use jacket or boiled potatoes and vegetables or salad of your choice.

Preparation and cooking time: 20 minutes
Serves: 2
1 tbsp plain flour
1/2 tsp paprika
1/2 tsp Cajun seasoning
1/2 tsp dried mixed herbs
Salt and pepper
2 skinless turkey breasts (weighing around 170g/6oz each)
2 tsp corn or rapeseed oil

1 Mix the flour with the paprika, Cajun seasoning, herbs, salt and pepper. Use this mixture to coat both sides of each turkey breast.
2 Heat the oil in a non-stick frying pan (skillet). Fry the turkey over a medium heat on both sides for about 15 minutes until the turkey is fully cooked.

Healthy Eating Notes

Turkey breast, like other poultry, is very low in fat. Choose it in preference to fatty meats and make sure you remove the skin and cook it with the minimum of added fat.

Fish dishes

Fish is today's convenience food – it is versatile, cooks quickly, comes in a variety of shapes and sizes and can be served in many different ways. As you'll see from the recipes in this chapter, fish blends well with a range of different flavours. Choose herbs such as parsley and dill, as in Cod in Parsley Sauce, or if you prefer a bit more spice, try Tandoori Prawns.

Countries where fish is eaten widely have low rates of heart disease. Scientific studies suggest that oily fish eaten regularly may give some protection against heart disease. The special 'omega-3' oils which come from fish have been shown to lower blood fats such as cholesterol. It is thought that omega-3 oils also help blood to flow more easily round the body by making it less sticky.

Oil-rich fish, such as mackerel, salmon and herring, are high in omega-3 oils. This type of fish is naturally moist and needs no added oil for basting or cooking; just use a little lemon juice. White fish, such as cod and plaice, are low in fat. However, all types of fish are a valuable source of protein and are low in saturated fat. Try to eat fish twice a week, with one of these choices being an oily fish.

Parchment-baked Cod

If serving this recipe at a dinner party, simply put the fish parcel on a plate and allow your guests to open it and release all the great aromas. Lemon and spring onions delicately flavour the fish without overpowering it. Wonderful with new potatoes in their jackets and steamed vegetables.

Preparation time: 5 minutes
Cooking time: 20 minutes
Serves: 4

- **4 x 175g/6oz cod fillets, skinned**
- **30g/1oz/¼ cup spring onions (scallions), chopped**
- **Juice and rind of 1 lemon**
- **Salt and freshly ground black pepper**

1 Preheat the oven to 200°C/400°F/Gas Mark 6.
2 Cut 4 squares of greaseproof (wax) paper, each approximately 30cm/ 12 inches square.
3 On each square place a fillet of cod, some spring onions, lemon rind and juice. Season to taste.
4 Make the greaseproof paper into parcels, sealing all the edges by using double folds.
5 Place each parcel on a large baking tray and bake for 20 minutes before serving.

Healthy Eating Notes

Cod is naturally low in fat and a good source of protein. In this recipe, no oil is necessary.

Cod in Parsley Sauce

Worried about lumpy sauces – or sticky washing up? This cheats' parsley sauce requires no cooking and yet has a wonderful creamy texture. Serve with boiled rice and salad, or new potatoes in their skins and vegetables.

Preparation time: 10 minutes
Cooking time: 20 minutes
Serves: 4

- **1 tbsp plain flour**
- **Salt and pepper**
- **4 cod fillets (weighing around 170g/6oz each)**
- **1 onion, finely chopped**
- **300g/10^1/$_2$oz can half-fat condensed mushroom soup**
- **3 tbsp lemon juice**
- **4 tbsp fresh parsley, chopped**
- **4 tomatoes, sliced**

1 Preheat the oven to 190°C/375°F/Gas Mark 5. Mix the flour with the seasoning and use this to coat each fillet.
2 Arrange the fish in a single layer at the bottom of a greased ovenproof dish.
3 Cover the fish with a layer of onion.
4 Mix the soup with the lemon juice and parsley. Pour this sauce over the fish and top with sliced tomatoes. Bake in the centre of the oven for 20 minutes till the fish is cooked.

Healthy Eating Notes

Choose fish in preference to fatty meats, and try to eat it twice a week. White fish such as cod is low in fat and ideal if you want to keep the calories down.

Trout Stuffed with Horseradish

Many people do not like bones with their fish – if this is the case, use trout fillets and roll them round the stuffing mixture, securing with a cocktail stick. Place in the greased foil and bake as directed.

Serve with new potatoes in their skins plus lightly cooked green beans.

Preparation time: 5 minutes
Cooking time: 25 minutes
Serves: 4

- **115g/4oz/^{2}/$_3$ cup fresh wholemeal breadcrumbs**
- **1 tbsp chopped parsley**
- **Finely grated rind and juice of 1 lemon**
- **Salt and pepper**
- **1 egg white**
- **30ml/2 tbsp horseradish sauce**
- **4 fresh trout (about 285g/10oz), gutted and cleaned**

1 Preheat the oven to 190°C/375°F/Gas Mark 5.
2 Make the stuffing by mixing the breadcrumbs, parsley, lemon juice and rind, seasoning, egg white and horseradish in a bowl.
3 Fill the cavities of the trout with the stuffing and wrap the fish in lightly greased foil.
4 Bake for 25 minutes.

Healthy Eating Notes

Cooking the fish in foil means that the rich fish oils provide moisture so there's no need to add extra.

Turkish Mackerel Wraps

This is great fun at a party – place all the food in the centre of the table and let your guests wrap their own!

Preparation time: 10 minutes
Cooking time: 10 minutes
Serves: 4

- 85g/3oz/$^1/_2$ cup carrot, grated
- 85g/3oz/$^1/_2$ cup red cabbage, finely shredded
- 40g/1$^1/_2$ oz/$^1/_4$ cup radish, finely sliced
- 4 fresh mackerel fillets (approx. 115g/4oz each), with no bones
- $^1/_2$ tsp ground cumin
- 8 tortilla wraps or Mediterranean bread (approx. 55g/2oz each)
- 2 lemons, halved

1 Preheat the grill (broiler) to high.
2 Mix together the grated carrot, red cabbage and radish in a bowl.
3 Sprinkle the ground cumin on the mackerel fillets and place on a large grill pan.
4 Grill the fish for 8–10 minutes, turning once.
5 Meanwhile, warm the bread then place a portion of the salad mixture in the centre.
6 When the mackerel is cooked, divide each fillet into two and place one on top of each salad and bread combination.
7 Wrap the salad and mackerel in the bread and serve with lemon halves to squeeze over.

Healthy Eating Notes

Mackerel is a rich source of omega-3 fatty acids, which are thought to be beneficial in preventing heart disease.

15-Minute Mackerel

Fresh orange juice helps to counteract the richness of this oily fish. Delicious with a large chunk of crusty bread and mixed salad, or boiled new potatoes in their skins and steamed mixed vegetables.

Preparation and cooking time: 15 minutes
Serves: 4

- **4 mackerel fillets (total weight around 395g/14oz)**
- **Juice of 2 fresh oranges**
- **1 clove garlic, crushed**
- **Salt and pepper**

1 Preheat the grill (broiler) to medium. Line the grill pan with foil and place each fillet skin side down on the foil.
2 Pour the orange juice over the mackerel and season with the garlic, salt and pepper.
3 Grill for 8–10 minutes, turning once after about 5 minutes.

Healthy Eating Notes

Although mackerel is high in fat, it is a good source of omega-3 fatty acids. Try to eat oily fish once a week.

Oatmeal Herrings

This recipe reminds me of my home town, Edinburgh. It is often served as part of a hearty Scottish breakfast. Accompany this rich fish with mashed or boiled potatoes and peas or broccoli.

Preparation and cooking time: 20 minutes
Serves: 4

- **115g/4oz/1¹/₃ cup oats**
- **Salt and pepper**
- **4 herrings, filleted**
- **1 tsp corn oil**
- **2 fresh lemons, sliced**

1 Mix the oats with a little salt and pepper. Coat both sides of each herring with the oats, pressing firmly onto the fish.
2 Heat the oil in a non-stick frying pan (skillet). Place the fish, two at a time, skin side upwards, into the pan. Fry over a high heat until the underside is lightly brown.
3 Turn the fish over and cook the other side. Remove from the pan.
4 Cook the other two fish in the same way.
5 Blot the fish on kitchen paper and serve with fresh lemon.

Healthy Eating Notes

The traditional way to cook herrings in Scotland is to fry them. Make sure you pat them with kitchen towel to remove the excess oil.

Halibut Fillets in White Wine

This goes well with basmati or wild rice and a lightly cooked green vegetable such as Peas with Shallots (*page 164*).

Preparation time: 5 minutes
Cooking time: 20 minutes
Serves: 4

- 10ml/2 tsp sunflower oil
- 1 large onion (approx. 225g/8oz), finely chopped
- 2 medium carrots (approx. 170g/6oz/1 cup), grated
- 1 can (395g/14oz/2 cups) chopped tomatoes
- 140ml/5fl oz/$^2/_3$ cup dry white wine
- 6 fresh basil leaves
- 30g/1oz chopped parsley
- 40g/1$^1/_2$ oz /$^1/_3$ cup spring onions (scallions), chopped
- 2 garlic cloves, crushed
- 565g/1$^1/_4$lb halibut fillets, skinned, boned and sliced thinly
- Salt and freshly ground black pepper

1 Heat the oil in a large, heavy-based frying pan (skillet).
2 Add the onion and cook until soft.
3 Stir in the carrots and cook for a further minute.
4 Add the chopped tomatoes, wine, basil leaves, chopped parsley, spring onions and garlic cloves.
5 Stir well and simmer for 5 minutes.
6 Add the fish, covering it with the tomato and vegetable mixture, and simmer over a low heat for 5 minutes.
7 Season the fish, turn it over and cook gently for a further 5 minutes before serving.

Healthy Eating Notes

This delicious recipe is low in fat.

Tuna and Sweetcorn Tagliatelle

Canned sweetcorn is very handy, but if you wish you could cook 2 corn cobs in boiling water for 10 minutes and then use the kernels scraped from the cob – this gives the dish a fresher taste. Some sweet red peppers are also a colourful addition. The yoghurt is used to give a creamy flavour, and a clever way to stop it curdling is to add some cornflour (cornstarch). This is delicious with a side dish of Minted Carrot Salad (*page 154*).

Preparation time: 5 minutes
Cooking time: 15 minutes
Serves: 4

- **300g/10¹/₂ oz/3¹/₂ cups tagliatelle**
- **15ml/1 tbsp olive oil**
- **1 large clove garlic, crushed**
- **140g/5oz/²/₃ cup natural yoghurt, mixed with 1 tsp cornflour (cornstarch)**
- **Juice of 1 lemon**
- **285g/10oz/1¹/₂ cups canned tuna in brine or spring water, drained**
- **255g/9oz/1¹/₄ cups canned sweetcorn in water, drained**
- **Freshly ground black pepper**
- **2 tbsp chopped parsley**

1 Cook the tagliatelle in boiling salted water until ready (normally about 10–12 minutes), then drain.
2 Heat the olive oil in a large pan and add the crushed garlic.
3 Stir in the natural yoghurt and lemon juice.
4 Mix in the cooked tagliatelle then add the drained tuna and sweetcorn.
5 Stir well to combine all the ingredients and heat thoroughly.
6 Add some freshly ground black pepper to taste and sprinkle with chopped parsley before turning out onto warmed serving plates.

Healthy Eating Notes

Pasta is nutritious and filling, with a low glycaemic index (*see Introduction*).

Tuna and Salsa Tortillas

Tortilla wraps are available from supermarkets, or you could pile the fillings into crispy taco shells instead.

Preparation time: 15 minutes
Serves: 4

For the filling
- **2 cans (185g/6¹/₂ oz/1 cup each) tuna in water, drained**
- **Juice of 1 lime**
- **¹/₂ tsp white wine vinegar**
- **Freshly ground black pepper**

For the salsa
- **30g/1oz/¹/₄ cup spring onions (scallions), chopped**
- **¹/₂ tsp garlic purée**
- **285g/10oz/1¹/₂ cups tomatoes, chopped**
- **¹/₂ tsp ground cumin**
- **Juice of 1 lime**
- **2 tbsp chopped parsley**
- **2 tbsp chopped coriander (cilantro)**
- **6 drops hot pepper sauce (optional)**
- **8 tortilla wraps (approx. 55g/2oz each)**
- **115g/4oz low-fat natural Greek yoghurt**

1 Make the salsa by combining all the ingredients in a bowl.
2 In another bowl, mash the tuna, lime juice and vinegar together and season with black pepper.
3 Warm the tortilla wraps in a microwave or under a hot grill (broiler).
4 To eat, place a warm tortilla on a plate. Top with a little salsa, yoghurt and tuna mixture and then wrap. Serve immediately.

Healthy Eating Notes
Choosing tuna canned in water or brine is a healthier alternative to oil.

Mussel and Smoked Haddock Stew

If you are not able to buy cooked mussels, you can easily boil them
yourself. Using some fish stock, boil them in their shells on a high heat
for 3 minutes. Discard any mussels whose shells have not opened.

Serve with either boiled rice or crusty bread and a green vegetable such
as mangetout or green beans.

Preparation time: 5 minutes
Cooking time: 15 minutes
Serves: 4

- **15ml/1 tbsp sunflower oil**
- **1 onion, finely chopped**
- **1 garlic clove, crushed**
- **455g/1lb/2^1/$_2$ cups smoked haddock fillets, skinned**
- **285ml/^{1}/$_2$ pint/1^1/$_3$ cups skimmed milk**
- **Sprigs of lemon thyme**
- **170g/6oz/1 cup mussels, cooked**
- **Pinch of saffron**
- **45ml/3 tbsp low-fat Greek yoghurt**

1 In a large saucepan, heat the oil then add the chopped onion and garlic.
2 Cook until soft, approximately 2 minutes.
3 Divide the smoked haddock into 4 pieces and lay on top of the onion
  mixture.
4 Add the milk and lemon thyme, bring to a gentle simmer and poach the
  haddock for 3 minutes.
5 Add the mussels and continue to cook for another 2 minutes.
6 With a slotted spoon, put the fish and mussels in heated bowls and
  keep warm.
7 Add the saffron to the milk mixture and boil for 3 minutes.
8 Reduce the heat and add the yoghurt, stirring to ensure it is well mixed.
9 Spoon over the fish and serve.

Healthy Eating Notes

The low-fat yoghurt makes a healthy alternative to cream. Remember that smoked fish is high in salt, so there's no need to add more!

Blackened Fish

Food from the Deep South of the United States has this classic blackened appearance. Blackened fish and chicken are becoming increasingly popular on restaurant menus in the UK. This recipe uses Cajun seasoning which is a unique blend of chillies, pepper, ginger and other spices. It comes ready mixed in a jar and you'll find it at the dried herbs counter in supermarkets.

The recipe needs virtually no preparation. Simply keep an eye on the pan and turn the fish a couple of times during cooking. Note that most bought frozen fish is usually best cooked from frozen. Check the label to see if defrosting is recommended.

Blackened fish goes well with boiled or baked potatoes or plain boiled rice. Remember to serve it with some vegetables – broccoli or French beans give a good contrasting colour.

Preparation and cooking time: 20 minutes
Serves: 2

- **1 tbsp oil**
- **1–2 tsp Cajun spice, as desired**
- **2 frozen haddock portions or fillets (weighing around 115g/4oz each)**

1 Heat the oil in a non-stick frying pan (skillet).
2 Sprinkle the Cajun spice liberally over one side of each piece of fish. Place the fish, seasoned side down, into the hot oil.
3 Sprinkle the top of the fish with the remaining Cajun spice. Turn the fish over after about 5 minutes. Cook the other side and turn again just to make sure the fish is cooked through. Serve immediately.

Healthy Eating Notes

Although it is best to cut down on fat and oil in cooking, you can pan-fry using very little oil. Choose oil high in unsaturated fat, such as olive, rapeseed or sunflower oils. Pat the fish with kitchen towel to remove excess oil.

Seafood Risotto

A risotto should have a thick, moist consistency – so make sure it is not too dry. If you want a vegetarian option, use vegetable stock and substitute the seafood with different vegetables like asparagus tips or wild mushrooms.

If using frozen seafood, ensure it is defrosted thoroughly in the fridge before use. Try this dish with some Cucumber and Mint Raita (*page 167*).

Preparation time: 5 minutes
Cooking time: 20 minutes
Serves: 4

- **15ml/1 tbsp olive oil**
- **2 red onions, finely chopped**
- **2 cloves garlic, crushed**
- **1 red chilli, chopped (optional)**
- **255g/9oz/1¼ cups risotto rice**
- **900ml/32fl oz/4 cups fish stock, heated**
- **395g/14oz/4 cups mixed seafood (mussels, prawns, scallops, squid)**
- **115g/4oz/²/₃ cup frozen petits pois**
- **Freshly ground black pepper**
- **Lemon and lime wedges (to garnish)**

1 Heat the oil in a large, heavy-based frying pan (skillet).
2 Add the onions and garlic (and red chilli if desired) and cook until soft.
3 Add the rice and cook for 2 minutes, stirring so that it is well coated.
4 Pour in ¼ of the heated stock and stir, waiting until it is absorbed before adding the next portion.
5 Stir regularly to prevent sticking, especially towards the end.
6 Cook the rice until *al dente* (approx. 20 minutes).
7 Add the seafood, frozen peas and some freshly ground black pepper and cook for a further 2 minutes until the fish and peas are thoroughly cooked. Ensure any prawns are a bright pink colour.
8 Serve garnished with lemon and lime wedges.

Healthy Eating Notes

Shellfish contain cholesterol, but this is not harmful to your blood cholesterol. This is because blood cholesterol is more influenced by the amount of saturated fat you eat.

Prawn Pilaff

A pilaff is an Eastern method of cooking rice with various spices. You can serve it alongside a main dish, as you would do with potatoes. Alternatively, it can be served as a main course if it is made with fish or chicken, as in this recipe. Although the list of spices in the ingredients may seem elaborate, you'll find they are very versatile and can be used to flavour leftovers. And this pilaff, surprisingly, takes only 15 minutes to prepare. Serve with some low-fat natural yoghurt dressing (such as Cucumber and Mint Raita, *see page 167*) and Tomato and Coriander Salad (*see page 155*).

Preparation time: 15 minutes
Cooking time: 20 minutes
Serves: 4

- **225g/8oz long-grain rice**
- **1 tbsp corn oil**
- **2 tsp cumin seeds**
- **2 tsp coriander (cilantro) seeds**
- **1 onion, sliced lengthways**
- **2 tsp crushed garlic (from a jar or tube)**
- **2 tomatoes, chopped**
- **$1/_2$ tsp turmeric**
- **$1/_4$ tsp salt**
- **170g/6oz fresh or frozen prawns, defrosted if necessary**
- **200g/7oz/$1^1/_2$ cups frozen peas**
- **500ml/18fl oz/$2^1/_4$ cups boiling water**

1 Rinse the rice and soak in plenty of cold water.
2 Heat the oil in a large non-stick pan with a lid. Add the cumin, coriander (cilantro), onion and garlic, and stir-fry for a few minutes to soften.
3 Add the tomatoes, turmeric and salt. Cook till the tomatoes are mushy, stirring occasionally.

4 Add the prawns and peas with the boiling water. Bring back to the boil, lower the heat, cover and simmer till the rice is cooked (about 15–20 minutes). All the water should be absorbed.

Healthy Eating Notes

Prawns are much lower in fat than meat and poultry.

Prawn Chow Mein

This quick and easy stir-fry looks impressive at a dinner party or is easy enough to prepare any day of the week. The noodles in this dish provide starchy carbohydrate.

Preparation and cooking time: 20 minutes
Serves: 4

- **2 tsp corn oil**
- **1 large onion, sliced lengthways**
- **1cm/^{1}/$_2$ inch root ginger, chopped or crushed**
- **200g/7oz/scant 2 cups fresh or frozen prawns, defrosted if necessary**
- **^{1}/$_4$ tsp Chinese five-spice powder**
- **115g/4oz/1^1/$_3$ cups beansprouts**
- **340g/11oz/1^1/$_2$ cups frozen sweetcorn, defrosted**
- **2 tbsp (30g/1oz) oyster sauce**
- **2 tbsp light soy sauce**
- **6 spring onions (scallions), sliced diagonally into 2cm/1-inch pieces**
- **225g/8oz thread egg noodles, cooked according to packet instructions**

1 Heat the oil in a wok or large pan. Stir-fry the onion and ginger for 2–3 minutes.
2 Add the prawns and five-spice powder and cook for a few minutes over a medium heat.
3 Stir in the beansprouts, sweetcorn, oyster sauce, soy sauce and spring onions (scallions) and cook for a further few minutes.
4 Mix in the noodles, adjust the seasoning and heat through.

Healthy Eating Notes

Prawns and shellfish contain cholesterol, but the cholesterol found in food does not have a significant effect on your blood cholesterol level. This is because blood cholesterol is more influenced by the amount of saturated fat in the diet and other factors, such as being overweight.

Tandoori Prawns

Tandoori dishes are familiar favourites in Indian restaurants where the food is cooked quickly in a very hot clay oven. In this recipe, the prawns are cooked over a high heat in tandoori spices, which are available in the herbs section in supermarkets.

The prawns are served in warmed wholemeal pitta bread filled with shredded lettuce. There's no need to add butter or spread because the tandoori sauce is quite moist. You may like to accompany this with more salad and some Cucumber and Mint Raita (*see page 167*).

Preparation and cooking time: 15 minutes
Serves: 2

- **2 tsp tandoori spice mix**
- **140g/5oz pot low-fat natural yoghurt**
- **1 tsp lemon juice**
- **225g/8oz/2 cups fresh or frozen prawns, defrosted if necessary**
- **1 tsp corn oil**
- **1 small onion, finely chopped**
- **2 tbsp chopped fresh coriander (cilantro)**
- **2 wholemeal pitta breads, warmed**
- **A few lettuce leaves, shredded**
- **1 fresh lemon, sliced**

1 Blend together the spice mix, yoghurt, lemon juice and prawns.
2 Heat the oil in a non-stick frying pan (skillet). Fry the onion over a medium heat until light brown.
3 Increase the heat to high and add the prawn mixture. Cook quickly, stirring frequently for about 5 minutes until the liquid is absorbed.
4 Stir in the coriander (cilantro) and remove from the heat.
5 Slit the pitta breads open and stuff them with the lettuce. Add the tandoori prawns and serve with lemon slices.

Healthy Eating Notes

Choose wholemeal pitta bread to provide more fibre. Using low-fat natural yoghurt in cooking helps to keep the overall fat content down.

Swordfish Kebabs

Swordfish is a really meaty fish that needs a strong-flavoured sauce to accompany it. It doesn't need to be summer to treat yourself to these kebabs on the barbecue – a grill (broiler) pan works just as well.

Preparation time: 15 minutes
Cooking time: 15 minutes
Serves: 4

- 70g/2$^{1}/_{2}$ oz baby corn
- 395g/14oz swordfish steaks, boned, skinned and cut into 1 cm/$^{1}/_{2}$-inch cubes
- 1 large red (bell) pepper
- 1 can (225g/8oz) water chestnuts in water, drained and halved

For the sauce
- 30ml/2 tbsp soy sauce
- 5ml/1 tsp rice wine vinegar
- Juice of 1 lemon
- $^{1}/_{2}$ tsp sugar
- $^{1}/_{2}$ tsp dried ginger powder

1 Cook the baby corn in boiling water for 3 minutes so it is soft but not easily broken.
2 Preheat the grill (broiler) to high.
3 Mix all the ingredients for the basting sauce together in a small dish.
4 Thread the swordfish, red pepper pieces, water chestnuts and baby corn onto 4 skewers.
5 Place on a large grill pan and baste thoroughly, turning to ensure they are coated on all sides. If there are any extra vegetables, put these on the grill pan too and baste with the sauce.
6 Place under a hot grill for 15 minutes, turning the kebabs to ensure they are fully cooked.

Healthy Eating Notes

The red pepper provides a valuable source of antioxidant vitamins.

Stir-fried Squid

Squid can be very tasty if cooked well. You will need to be careful not to overcook the squid or it will become rubbery and chewy in texture. Serve with plain boiled egg noodles and some grilled red peppers for a colourful and tasty meal.

Preparation and cooking time: 20 minutes
Serves: 4

- **30g/1oz plain (all purpose) flour**
- **Salt and freshly ground black pepper**
- **340g/12oz/3 cups fresh squid rings**
- **15ml/1 tbsp sunflower oil**
- **1 stalk lemon grass, finely shredded**
- **1 red chilli, seeds removed and cut finely**
- **115g/4oz/4 cups watercress, washed**

1 Season the flour with salt and pepper and toss the squid rings to coat them.
2 In a wok, heat the oil to a high temperature.
3 Add the squid, lemon grass and chilli and stir-fry for 3 minutes, stirring to prevent sticking.
4 Add the watercress and continue to cook for a further 3 minutes until the watercress is wilted and the squid is cooked.

Healthy Eating Notes

Watercress is a good source of iron.

Hot Potato and Anchovy Salad

Marinated anchovies are available from the delicatessen counter or can be bought vacuum packed. Do not use the bottled variety for this recipe as they are too strong and salty.

Preparation and cooking time: 25 minutes
Serves: 4

- **500g/18oz/3¹/₂ cups baby new potatoes (a waxy type such as Carlingford is best)**
- **2 red (bell) peppers (170g/6oz/1¹/₂ cups each), seeded and sliced**
- **115g/4oz/1 cup marinated anchovies, drained (reserve the liquid)**
- **55g/2oz/¹/₂ cup spring onions (scallions), trimmed and chopped**
- **1 tsp dried tomatoes, finely chopped**

1 Boil the new potatoes for approximately 20 minutes until tender.
2 Meanwhile, place the sliced red peppers on a baking tray and grill (broil) under a high heat until they start to blacken.
3 In a large bowl, mix the drained anchovies, spring onions and dried tomatoes.
4 Add the grilled peppers when ready.
5 Drain the potatoes and shake in the pan to roughen the surfaces (don't shake too much or they will disintegrate!).
6 Add to the salad while still hot and pour over 2 tsp of the oil/vinegar/herb mixture reserved from the anchovies.
7 Mix thoroughly and serve.

Healthy Eating Notes

The potatoes are naturally low in fat and help to fill you up.

Pilchard Pastries

Pilchards are extremely economical and if you don't like the distinctive smell of fish, mixing the pilchards with mushrooms and cheese helps to remove this.

Preparation and cooking time: 30 minutes
Serves: 4

- 115g/4oz/1 cup onions, finely chopped
- 85g/3oz/1 cup mushrooms, finely chopped
- 15ml/1 tbsp sunflower oil
- 1 can (425g/15oz/2¹/₂ cups) pilchards in brine, drained and bones removed
- 55g/2oz/¹/₃ cup cottage cheese
- 15g/¹/₂ oz/1 tbsp tomato purée (paste)
- 8 sheets filo pastry (approx. 12 x 20cm/5 x 8 inches each)
- 30ml/1fl oz skimmed milk
- Lemon wedges (to garnish)
- Fresh parsley (to garnish)

1 Preheat the oven to 190°C/375°F/Gas Mark 5.
2 In a heavy-based frying pan (skillet), fry the chopped onions and mushrooms in 2 tsp sunflower oil until soft.
3 Mix in the pilchards, cottage cheese and tomato purée and ensure it is well blended.
4 Take 2 sheets of filo pastry together and place ¹/₄ of the fish mixture in one corner.
5 Fold the filo pastry around the mixture, making a large triangle. Seal all the pastry joins with water.
6 Place on a baking tray and repeat the process for the other 3 triangles.
7 Brush with skimmed milk and bake for 10 minutes.
8 Remove and brush with the remaining tsp of oil and bake for a further 5–10 minutes until brown.
9 Serve garnished with lemon triangles and parsley.

Healthy Eating Notes

Ready-made filo pastry is easy to use and does not have the heavy fat or calorie content of most pastry.

Jumbo Salmon Fish Cakes

Serve these hot with baked beans or with a salad and home-made Salsa Sauce (*see page 166*).

Preparation time: 25 minutes
Cooking time: 10 minutes
Makes: 6

- 125g/4$^{1}/_{2}$oz packet instant mashed potato mix
- 225g/8oz canned red salmon
- 2 tbsp chopped fresh dill
- 1 tbsp lemon juice
- Salt and pepper
- 1 tbsp corn oil, plus a little for greasing
- 1 egg, beaten
- 115g/4oz cornflakes, crushed

1 Preheat the grill (broiler) to high.
2 Make up the mashed potato according to the instructions on the packet. Mix in the salmon, dill, lemon juice and seasoning.
3 Divide the mixture into six portions and form each portion into a fish cake.
4 Line the grill pan with foil and brush some oil over the foil.
5 Dip each fish cake into the beaten egg and then into the crushed cornflakes.
6 Arrange the coated fish cakes on the greased foil.
7 Drizzle the remaining tablespoon of oil over the fish cakes. Grill (broil) for 10 minutes, turning once halfway through cooking.

Healthy Eating Notes

Fish cakes are usually fried. Even shallow frying will make the fish cakes absorb far more fat than that used in this recipe. For a higher-fibre recipe, you can use wholemeal breadcrumbs or bran-flakes instead of the cornflakes.

Salmon in Cream and Mustard Sauce

A special dish for entertaining and dinner parties made from lightly poached salmon and half-fat crème fraîche. Serve with boiled new potatoes and vegetables. Delicious with whole French beans and carrots.

Preparation and cooking time: 20 minutes
Serves: 4

- **600g/21oz salmon fillet, cut into 4 portions**
- **A few sprigs fresh parsley**
- **1 bay leaf**
- **3 tbsp lemon juice**
- **6 peppercorns**

For the sauce
- **170g/6oz half-fat crème fraîche**
- **1 tsp coarse-grain mustard**
- **2 tbsp fresh chopped dill or 1 tsp dried dill weed**
- **Salt and coarsely ground black pepper**
- **1 fresh lemon, quartered**

1 Place the fish, parsley, bay leaf, lemon juice and peppercorns in lightly salted boiling water. Bring to the boil and simmer for about 10–12 minutes or until the fish flakes when tested with a fork.
2 Lift out the cooked fish with a slotted spoon.
3 Strain the liquid and add 4 tbsp to the crème fraîche. Put into a frying pan (skillet) and heat gently till boiling. Add the mustard, dill and seasoning. Heat through and pour the sauce over the fish. Serve with fresh lemon.

Healthy Eating Notes

Dairy products are everyday foods, so choosing lower-fat versions can help you cut down on fat. Examples are reduced-fat spread, reduced-fat cheese, skimmed and semi-skimmed milk and low-fat yoghurt.

Vegetarian dishes

If you're about to flick past this chapter because you're not vegetarian, then STOP! These recipes will introduce you to a wide variety of pulses and pastas as well as unusual ways of serving up vegetables. You can make a main meal of these nutritious dishes or simply team them up with meat or fish. And there's no need to soak dried pulses or do lots of chopping up and preparation. Serve up Caribbean Rice or Pasta Shells with Olives and Oregano in less than 30 minutes.

Vegetarian dishes can be healthier, but this isn't always so, because dishes based on eggs and cheese can be high in fat. This chapter will show you how to choose reduced-fat versions of standard ingredients with no compromise on taste.

Recipes in this book have been specifically designed to cater for people who have diabetes or who wish to eat more healthily. If you are vegetarian, pulse vegetables such as beans and lentils provide a valuable source of protein. Together with starchy foods such as rice and pasta, you can prepare perfectly balanced meals. Pasta is particularly beneficial in diabetes because it has a more gradual effect on your blood glucose levels than many other carbohydrates.

A diet that contains plenty of fruit and vegetables is associated with a reduced risk of heart disease and cancer. Beans and pulses are an excellent source of soluble fibre, which has been shown to lower blood cholesterol. What's more, vegetables contain the antioxidant vitamins betacarotene and vitamin C, which are also protective against heart disease. All in all, vegetables are foods we should be eating more of. Use the recipes in this section to help you select the recommended amount of two large helpings of vegetables each day.

Chunky Hummus Topped with Grilled Vegetables

Serve with warm pitta bread, either as a starter or a lunchtime treat.

Preparation time: 15 minutes
Cooking time: 10 minutes
Serves: 4

For the hummus
- **1 can (395g/14oz/1$\frac{1}{2}$ cups) chickpeas in water, drained (but reserve liquid)**
- **2 cloves garlic, peeled**
- **Juice of 2 lemons**
- **55g/2oz/4 tbsp tahini (sesame seed paste)**

For the grilled vegetables
- **115g/4oz/1 cup aubergine (eggplant), thinly sliced**
- **115g/4oz/1 cup courgette (zucchini), thinly sliced**
- **1 red (bell) pepper, stalk and seeds removed, quartered**
- **1 yellow/orange (bell) pepper, stalk and seeds removed, quartered**
- **5ml/1 tsp olive oil**

To serve
- **10ml/2 tsp olive oil**
- **Paprika, for sprinkling**

1 Preheat the grill (broiler) to hot. Make the hummus by blending all the ingredients together in a liquidiser with approximately 60ml/2fl oz/ $\frac{1}{4}$ cup reserved chickpea liquid. Do not make it too smooth! Chill in the refrigerator.
2 Meanwhile, lay the vegetables on a large baking tray and brush with the olive oil.
3 Cook under a hot grill for 10 minutes, turning once.
4 To serve, place a mound of hummus on a large dinner plate and lay the grilled vegetables over the top. Drizzle with the olive oil and sprinkle with a little paprika.

Healthy Eating Notes

Chickpeas have a wonderful flavour and are a rich source of soluble fibre. A portion of pulses counts towards your 'five a day' target of fruit and vegetables, and this canned variety is fine as part of a varied diet.

Lentil and Vegetable Combo

This healthy combination is tasty on top of jacket potatoes or wrapped in tortillas. If you like a bit of spice, you could add a chopped red chilli too. Do not add salt to the liquid when boiling the lentils as this will delay the cooking process.

Preparation time: 10 minutes
Cooking time: 15 minutes
Serves: 4

- 115g/4oz/$^1/_2$ cup red lentils
- 200ml/7fl oz/$^3/_4$ cup vegetable stock
- 15ml/1 tbsp sunflower oil
- 140g/5oz/$^3/_4$ cup carrot, grated
- 1 large onion (225g/8 oz/2 cups), diced
- 1 green pepper (170g/6oz/1$^1/_2$ cups), diced
- 115g/4oz/$^2/_3$ cup tomatoes, diced
- 1 large cooking apple (395g/14oz/3 cups), peeled, cored and grated
- 2 cloves garlic, crushed
- 1 tbsp chopped fresh sage
- 30g/1oz/$^1/_5$ cup raisins
- 55g/2oz/$^1/_3$ cup unsalted peanuts
- 115g/4oz/$^1/_2$ cup low-fat soft cheese

1. Simmer the red lentils in the vegetable stock until soft (approx. 8–10 minutes), then drain.
2. Meanwhile, heat the sunflower oil in a large frying pan (skillet) and add the grated carrots, onion, green pepper, tomatoes, grated apple, garlic and sage.
3. Mix and then cook for 15 minutes.
4. Add the lentils, raisins and peanuts and stir in the low-fat soft cheese.
5. Heat thoroughly then serve.

Healthy Eating Notes

Lentils provide an excellent source of protein in a vegetarian diet.

Lentil Burgers with Limed Tomato Sauce

Canned green lentils are widely available in most large supermarkets and are ideal for this recipe. Greenish-brown and slightly peppery in flavour, they marry well with the potato and onion. They can be made well in advance, if you like, but flour them at the last minute before you start cooking.

Preparation time: 15 minutes
Cooking time: 15 minutes
Serves: 4

- 115g/4oz/1 cup onion, very finely chopped
- 215g/7^1/$_2$oz/1^1/$_2$ cups made-up instant mashed potato (made from 40g/1^1/$_2$oz/3 tbsp dried potato powder)
- 500g/18oz/just over 2^1/$_2$ cups (drained and rinsed weight) canned green lentils
- 15g/^{1}/$_2$oz/1 tbsp freshly chopped coriander (cilantro)
- Salt and freshly ground black pepper
- 30g/1oz/^{2}/$_3$ cup flour
- 15ml/^{1}/$_2$oz/1 tbsp olive oil

For the sauce
- 225g/8oz/^{3}/$_4$ cup passata
- 15ml/1 tbsp fresh lime juice
- 2–3 drops hot pepper sauce (e.g. Tabasco) or to taste
- 1 tsp caster sugar

1 Mix the onion with the mashed potatoes.
2 Put the lentils into a blender or food processor and whiz for a few seconds until smooth.
3 Add the puréed lentils to the potato mixture. Season to taste with the coriander and black pepper.
4 Form into 4 burgers.
5 Coat lightly with flour and shallow-fry in the hot olive oil for 5 minutes on each side until heated through.

6 Combine the ingredients for the sauce, heat through and serve over the burgers.

Healthy Eating Notes

These burgers are much lower in fat than beef burgers and contain a valuable source of protein in the lentils.

Warm Lentil Salad with Sunshine Vegetables

Canned green lentils tend to look a bit drab on their own, but this salad is a lovely riot of colour – wonderful red, yellow and green peppers, sweet 'n' succulent cherry tomatoes, chopped spring onions and fragrant fresh basil. It's also very quick and simple to prepare.

Preparation time: 15 minutes
Cooking time: 5 minutes
Serves: 4

- 15ml/1 tbsp olive oil
- 55g/2oz/$^1/_2$ cup spring onions (scallions), chopped
- 170g/6oz/1$^1/_2$ cups each sliced red, yellow and green (bell) peppers
- 500g/18oz/just over 2$^1/_2$ cups (drained and rinsed weight) canned green lentils
- 225g/8oz cherry tomatoes, halved
- 45ml/3 tbsp oil-free French dressing
- 15g/$^1/_2$oz/$^1/_2$ cup fresh basil leaves (to garnish)

1 Heat the olive oil in a large, non-stick frying pan (skillet) or wok (a wok is better), and stir-fry the spring onions and peppers for 2 minutes.
2 Add the lentils and warm through.
3 Lightly mix in the cherry tomatoes, add the French dressing and give the whole mixture a good toss.
4 Turn into a salad bowl and serve, still warm, garnished with the fresh basil leaves.

Healthy Eating Notes

This recipe is packed with vegetables, helping you to eat your recommended amount of at least two large portions per day. The lentils provide an excellent source of protein and soluble fibre.

Grilled Avocado and Hazelnuts

This recipe could easily be baked in the oven, but it would take slightly longer to prepare. It is worth finding fresh lemon grass and chopping it very finely as this imparts an aromatic lemon flavour that nothing else really matches. Serve with a mixed salad and some crusty bread.

Preparation time: 15 minutes
Cooking time: 5 minutes
Serves: 4

- 85g/3oz/^{2}/$_3$ cup red onion, diced
- 5ml/1 tsp olive oil
- 85g/3oz/1 cup ground hazelnuts
- 15g/^{1}/$_2$ oz parsley, chopped
- 2 stalks lemon grass, very finely chopped
- 2 ripe avocado pears
- 15g/^{1}/$_2$oz/^{1}/$_4$ cup Parmesan cheese, finely grated

1 Preheat the grill (broiler) to medium.
2 Place the red onion in a pan with the olive oil and cook until soft (approximately 3 minutes).
3 In a bowl, mix together the ground hazelnuts, chopped parsley and lemon grass and the cooked onion.
4 Prepare the avocados by cutting in half and removing the stone. Remove a fine sliver of skin from the bases so the avocados will sit firmly and not fall over.
5 Remove the flesh from the avocados and mash into the nut mixture.
6 Pile the mixture back into the avocados and cover with Parmesan cheese.
7 Flash under the grill until hot, but be careful that the cheese or hazelnuts do not burn.

Healthy Eating Notes

Nuts are an excellent source of protein. Both hazelnuts and avocados are rich in fat, but the good news is that it's monounsaturated fat.

Savoury Ratatouille Pancakes

As well as using this ratatouille as a filling for pancakes, you could also serve it with crusty bread, veggie sausages, nut loaf or to top a jacket potato. It is also wonderful served cold as a side salad.

The pancakes are fairly thick to hold the filling, but if you prefer a thinner version, simply add more milk to the recipe.

Preparation time: 15 minutes
Cooking time: 15 minutes
Serves: 4

For the ratatouille filling
- **2 tsp olive oil**
- **1 large onion (200g/7oz/2 cups), chopped**
- **2–3 cloves garlic, crushed**
- **285g/10oz/2^1/$_2$ cups aubergine (eggplant), cut into bite-sized dice**
- **285g/10oz/2^1/$_2$ cups courgette (zucchini), cut into bite-sized dice**
- **200g/7oz/2 cups red (bell) pepper, sliced**
- **310g/11oz/1^1/$_3$ cups passata**

For the pancakes
- **115g/4oz/^{2}/$_3$ cup plain (all purpose) wholemeal flour**
- **Pinch of salt**
- **100ml/3^1/$_2$fl oz/^{1}/$_2$ cup skimmed milk**
- **2 eggs**
- **10ml/2 tsp sunflower oil**

1 In a large saucepan, heat the oil and add the onion and garlic.
2 Cook until soft but not brown (approximately 5 minutes).
3 Add the aubergine, courgette and red pepper and cook, covered, for a further 10 minutes. Make the pancake batter (see step 5).
4 Add the passata and simmer until ready to serve.
5 Make the pancake batter at stage 3, above.
6 Add the milk to the flour and salt then beat in the eggs.

7   Spray a small pancake pan with a little sunflower oil, heat to a high temperature and add $1/8$ of the batter mixture.

8   Tilt it to spread the batter mixture and cook until the small bubbles in the mixture have started to burst.

9   Flip the pancake and cook for another 30 seconds to ensure the second side is cooked.

10   Place in foil to keep warm while you make the rest of the pancakes.

11   Serve with the ratatouille mixture spilling out of the folded pancakes.

Healthy Eating Notes

This recipe is packed with vegetables, helping you to eat the recommended amount of at least two large portions a day.

Fresh Herb Couscous

A fresh-tasting but simple dish to accompany grilled vegetable kebabs. It also goes well with Turkey Fricassee (*page 75*). Throw in a can of red kidney beans if you want something more filling.

Preparation time: 15 minutes
Cooking time: 15 minutes
Serves: 4

- 140g/5oz/$^2/_3$ cup couscous
- 230ml/8fl oz /1 cup hot vegetable stock
- 55g/2oz/$^1/_2$ cup spring onions (scallions), chopped
- 55g/2oz/$^1/_2$ cup flat-leaf parsley, chopped
- 55g/2oz/$^1/_2$ cup coriander (cilantro) leaves, chopped
- 200g/7oz/1 cup tomatoes, chopped into small dice
- Juice of 4 lemons
- 10ml/2 tsp olive oil

1 Put the couscous in a large bowl and pour over the hot stock.
2 Mix once with a fork and leave to stand for 5 minutes.
3 Add the remaining ingredients and mix well.
4 Leave to stand for a further 10 minutes for the flavours to blend.

Healthy Eating Notes

Seasoning with herbs instead of salt is a healthier option. Too much salt can raise blood pressure.

Noodles with Pesto and Mango

With a slightly sweet and sour flavour, these noodles can definitely be eaten on their own. They also go well mixed with grilled tofu or your favourite stir-fry. This amount makes two large portions or three medium servings.

Preparation time: 5 minutes
Cooking time: 5 minutes
Serves: 2–3

- **30g/1oz pine nuts**
- **140g/5oz/1 cup Chinese medium egg noodles, dried**
- **1 can (425g/15oz/2 cups) mango pieces tinned in natural juice, drained or 1 large fresh mango, stone removed, sliced and peeled**
- **30g/1oz pesto sauce**
- **Freshly ground black pepper**
- **Basil leaves (to garnish)**

1 Preheat the grill (broiler) to high.
2 Place the pine nuts on a baking tray and toast under the grill until light brown, shaking continuously to prevent burning.
3 Put the noodles in a pan of boiling water, stir and turn off the heat. Leave for 3 minutes and then drain.
4 In a large pan over a low heat, mix together the cooked noodles, toasted pine nuts, mango pieces and pesto until hot.
5 Season with black pepper and sprinkle with basil leaves before serving.

Healthy Eating notes

Noodles are a good source of valuable carbohydrate.

Apple Caesar Salad

Caesar salad is one of the most calorific salads you can have, so it's not an everyday dish. This recipe uses lower-fat ingredients so you will be a little more virtuous, but still go easy on how often you indulge … it's finger-licking good!

Preparation time: 20 minutes (add an extra 10 minutes if you are making the dressing from scratch)
Serves: 4

- 140g/5oz French bread slices
- 5ml/1 tsp olive oil
- 140g/5oz/2 cups cos or romaine lettuce, roughly torn
- 255g/9oz/2 cups red apples, cored and sliced (but not peeled), mixed with the juice of 1 lemon
- 55g/2oz/$^{1}/_{2}$ cup walnut pieces
- 15g/$^{1}/_{2}$oz/$^{1}/_{4}$ cup Parmesan cheese, grated roughly into shavings
- 2 tbsp reduced-fat Caesar dressing, either shop-bought or see below

1 Preheat the oven to 230°C/450°F/Gas Mark 8.
2 Place the French bread slices on a baking tray and brush with the olive oil on both sides.
3 Cook in the oven for 10 minutes until crispy.
4 Meanwhile, place the lettuce in a large salad bowl.
5 Drain the apple slices of any excess lemon juice then add to the lettuce with the walnut pieces and cheese.
6 When the bread is crispy, remove from the oven and cut into croutons.
7 Sprinkle over the salad and mix well.
8 Add the salad dressing and toss before serving.

Home-made Reduced-fat Caesar Dressing

Makes: 8 servings

- **1 egg yolk**
- **1 clove garlic, pressed**
- **10ml/2 tsp white wine vinegar**
- **5ml/1 tsp lemon juice**
- **1 tsp Dijon mustard**
- **30ml/2 tbsp olive oil**
- **30ml/2 tbsp low-fat natural yoghurt**
- **Salt and freshly ground black pepper**

1 Simply whisk all the ingredients together well.

Healthy Eating Notes

A reduced-fat dressing makes this salad a much healthier option. The apple contributes to your recommended daily intake of fruit.

Strawberry and Walnut Salad

This combination of colourful vegetables with strawberries and tarragon makes a stunning salad that would be suitable for either entertaining or a cosy lunch for two.

Preparation time: 15 minutes
Standing time: 10 minutes
Serves: 4

- 200g/7oz/1¹/₄ cups tomatoes, thinly sliced
- 70g/2¹/₂oz/¹/₂ cup spring onions (scallions), cut as instructed below
- 70g/2¹/₂oz/¹/₂ cup radishes, thinly sliced
- 115g/4oz/²/₃ cup strawberries, trimmed and thinly sliced
- 1¹/₂ tsp fresh tarragon, finely chopped
- Freshly ground salt and black pepper
- 2cm/1-inch chunk of cucumber, finely sliced
- 1 tsp chopped walnuts
- 15ml/1 tbsp walnut oil

1 Lay the thinly sliced tomatoes as a bottom layer on a large plate.
2 Cut the green section of the spring onions into 1cm/¹/₂-inch lengths and slice the white bulb finely.
3 Lay over the tomatoes, followed by the radish then the strawberry slices.
4 Sprinkle over the fresh tarragon and season with freshly ground salt and black pepper.
5 Lay the sliced cucumber on top, sprinkle with the chopped walnuts and drizzle over the walnut oil, ensuring it reaches the layers below.
6 The salad benefits from standing for about 10 minutes at room temperature for the flavours to blend.

Healthy Eating Notes

Bursting with vitamins C and E, this recipe has the bonus of being low in fat.

Vegetable Chilli

This differs from traditional chilli con carne in two ways – first, obviously, it doesn't contain any meat. Second, the rice is incorporated in the dish, rather than being served separately, making it more in the style of a vegetarian paella or risotto. And this means that the rice absorbs all the delicious flavours of the vegetables.

Preparation time: 10 minutes
Cooking time: 15–20 minutes
Serves: 4

- **15ml/1 tbsp garlic-flavoured olive oil**
- **115g/4oz/1 cup chopped onion or leek (you can use either)**
- **115g/4oz/1 cup each red and green (bell) peppers, coarsely diced**
- **2 tsp ground turmeric**
- **300g/10¹/₂ oz/1¹/₂ cups long-grain rice**
- **5ml/1 tsp hot pepper sauce (such as Tabasco)**
- **700ml/1¹/₄ pints/2³/₄ cups hot vegetable stock (from 2 cubes)**
- **340g/12oz/2 cups (drained weight) canned red kidney beans**
- **Freshly ground black pepper**
- **15g/1oz/¹/₄ cup freshly chopped coriander (cilantro) (to garnish)**

1 Heat the olive oil in a large, non-stick pan or a wok (a wok is better for sautéing the vegetables).
2 Quickly stir-fry the onion or leek and peppers for 1 minute.
3 Add the turmeric, give the pan another quick stir, then stir in the rice and hot pepper sauce. Mix thoroughly.
4 Stir in the hot vegetable stock and bring quickly to the boil.
5 Lower the heat, cover and simmer for 12 minutes or until the rice is tender and all the liquid is absorbed. (Check after about 10 minutes and, if the mixture gets too dry, add a little hot water.)
6 Mix in the kidney beans, heat for another minute and season to taste with black pepper.
7 Serve garnished with the fresh coriander.

Healthy Eating Notes

The beans provide a good source of fibre and protein, and whole beans have a low glycaemic index.

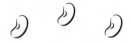

Caribbean Rice

A one-pot dish that needs 10 minutes of your time and is then left to cook completely on its own. Add the chillies according to your taste. If you prefer dishes with a bit more spice, choose hot Jamaican chilli peppers or Jamaican jerk seasoning, which are available in West Indian grocery shops. Use this recipe to add a starchy accompaniment to your main dish, or serve it as a main meal with a fresh side salad, such as Tomato and Coriander Salad (*see page 155*).

Preparation time: 10 minutes
Cooking time: 20 minutes
Serves: 4

- **1 tbsp corn oil**
- **1 onion, finely chopped**
- **170g/6oz/³/₄ cup canned chopped tomatoes in tomato juice**
- **2 fresh green chillies, chopped or 2 tsp chilli sauce**
- **Salt and pepper**
- **425g/15oz can pigeon peas or red kidney beans, drained**
- **225g/8oz/1 heaping cup rice**
- **500ml/18fl oz/2¹/₄ cups boiling water**

1 Heat the oil in a large saucepan with a lid. Fry the onion until browned (about 5 minutes).
2 Add the tomatoes, chillies and seasoning. Cook for a few minutes.
3 Gently stir in the peas (or beans), rice and boiling water.
4 Bring back to the boil, lower the heat, cover and cook for about 20 minutes until all the water is absorbed.

Healthy Eating Notes

You do not need to use brown rice in this recipe since there is already extra fibre in the added vegetables.

Vegetable Rice

Delicious with some crisp salad dressed with fat-free vinaigrette.

Preparation time: 10 minutes
Cooking time: 20 minutes
Serves: 4

- **1 tbsp corn oil**
- **1 onion, finely chopped**
- **2 vegetable stock cubes, made up to 500ml/18fl oz/2¼ cups with boiling water**
- **225g/8oz/1 heaping cup long-grain rice**
- **455g/1lb frozen mixed vegetables**
- **¹/₂ tsp ground turmeric**
- **Salt and pepper**

1 Heat the oil in a large saucepan with a lid. Fry the onion until browned (about 5 minutes).
2 Add all the other ingredients.
3 Bring back to the boil, lower the heat, cover and cook for about 20 minutes until all the water is absorbed.

Healthy Eating Notes

Vegetables and starchy foods together can make well-balanced, low-calorie meals.

Mexican Butter Beans with Rice

An unusual dish made from rice and vegetables – a perfect vegetarian meal with no need for any accompaniments.

Preparation and cooking time: 20 minutes
Serves: 2

- **115g/4oz/2 cups long-grain rice, freshly cooked**
- **140g/5oz/³/₄ cup canned butter beans, drained**
- **2 tsp oil**
- **1 onion, finely chopped**
- **1 clove garlic, crushed (optional)**
- **1 green (bell) pepper, diced**
- **1 tsp red chilli powder, or to taste**
- **115g/4oz/¹/₂ cup chopped tinned tomatoes**
- **85g/3oz low-fat soft cheese**
- **2 tbsp chopped fresh coriander (cilantro)**

1 Preheat the grill (broiler) to medium.
2 Lightly grease a flameproof dish and place the cooked rice into this dish.
3 Put the beans on top of the rice.
4 Heat the oil and fry the onion, garlic (if used) and pepper. Cook for a few minutes to soften them.
5 Add the chilli and tomatoes and cook till the mixture becomes mushy.
6 Stir in the soft cheese and cover the beans with this sauce. Add most of the coriander (cilantro), saving a little for garnish.
7 Grill (broil) for about a minute, garnish and serve immediately.

Healthy Eating Notes

Beans and rice both contain protein, and serving them together like this helps to provide a balanced meal. All beans and lentils are rich in protein and soluble fibre and are low in fat.

Fresh Tagliatelle with Blue Cheese and Walnut Sauce

Danish blue cheese has an intense flavour so you don't need to use much. You can use any other fresh pasta, as long as it's not filled, but hollow varieties such as macaroni and pasta shells will soak up much more of the sauce and may make the dish rather dry. The recipe itself is child's play, and very quick.

Preparation time: 5 minutes
Cooking time: 10 minutes
Serves: 4

- 570ml/^{1}/$_2$ pint/1^1/$_4$ cups half-fat crème fraîche
- ^{1}/$_4$ pint/^{1}/$_2$ cup
- 55g/2oz Danish blue cheese
- Salt and white pepper to taste
- 115g/4oz/1 cup walnut pieces
- 500g/18oz fresh tagliatelle or pasta of choice

1 Put a large pan of salted water on to boil.
2 Put the crème fraîche into another saucepan and crumble in the blue cheese.
3 Warm gently and stir until the cheese has melted, season to taste with salt and white pepper and crumble in the walnut pieces.
4 When the water is boiling, throw in the pasta and cook for about 4 minutes or until done to your liking. If you prefer a more saucey pasta, add some more skimmed milk and stir well at this point.
5 Drain well and serve with the hot sauce.

Healthy Eating Notes
The half-fat crème fraîche and skimmed milk help keep the fat content down.

Pasta Shells with Olives and Oregano

A large portion lasts for days when your eyes are bigger than your stomach! This Italian meal needs only a side salad and bread to make it complete.

Preparation and cooking time: 20 minutes
Serves: 3

- 255g/8oz/2²/₃ cups pasta shells
- 1 tbsp olive oil
- 2 cloves garlic, crushed
- 1 onion, finely chopped
- 1 green (bell) pepper, diced
- 1¹/₂ tsp dried oregano
- 55g/2oz pitted black olives
- Salt and coarsely ground black pepper

1 Cook the pasta in lightly salted water according to the instructions on the packet.
2 Meanwhile, heat the oil in a large non-stick pan. Add the garlic, onion and green (bell) pepper and fry until the onion is light brown and the pepper just cooked (about 5–7 minutes).
3 Stir in the oregano, olives, pasta and seasoning, and serve.

Healthy Eating Notes

Raw vegetables contain more vitamin C than cooked. Try to cook vegetables quickly in the minimum of water so you retain as much of the vitamins as possible.

Macaroni and Cauliflower Cheese

Frozen cauliflower florets and an instant sauce sachet help to make this into a substantial, quick and easy meal. Choose a sauce mix to which you add milk, not water. This way you can use skimmed milk to help keep the fat down. If you can only find a sauce which is made up with boiling water, then bear in mind that the fat content may be a little higher. This is because the sauce mix may have been made with full-fat milk or added fat. Serve with vegetables such as broccoli, spinach or peas.

Preparation and cooking time: 35 minutes
Serves: 4

- **225g/8oz macaroni**
- **395g/14oz/3$^{1}/_{2}$ cups frozen cauliflower florets**
- **20g/$^{3}/_{4}$oz packet instant white sauce mix**
- **285ml/$^{1}/_{2}$ pint/1$^{1}/_{3}$ cups skimmed milk**
- **115g/4oz/1 cup half-fat Cheddar cheese, grated**
- **Salt and pepper**
- **$^{1}/_{2}$ tsp French mustard**
- **2 tomatoes, sliced (optional)**

1 Cook the macaroni according to the instructions on the packet.
2 Meanwhile, steam or boil the cauliflower until just cooked.
3 Follow the instructions for making up the sauce, using the skimmed milk if required.
4 Stir in most of the cheese and season the sauce with the salt, pepper and mustard.
5 Preheat the grill (broiler) to medium.
6 Mix the cooked, drained macaroni into the sauce and adjust the seasoning if necessary.
7 Put the mixture into a lightly greased flameproof dish. Sprinkle the remaining cheese and the sliced tomatoes on top. Grill (broil) until the cheese is brown and bubbling.

Healthy Eating Notes

Using skimmed milk and half-fat cheese makes this dish lower in fat than traditional recipes. If you don't like the taste of half- or reduced-fat cheeses, use a small amount of stronger-flavoured full-fat cheese. Low-fat alternatives can help you to reduce your fat intake as long as you don't eat more of them than your usual brand.

Vegetable Pasta in Tomato Sauce

I usually use pasta spirals or penne for this recipe. The pasta is not coated in a thick tomato sauce, but has just the right amount of tomato flavour and a hint of garlic. This is a dish you can serve on its own, especially since pasta is so filling. If anything, a side salad is all you need.

Preparation and cooking time: 30 minutes
Serves: 4

* **285g/10oz/3 cups pasta**
* **1 tbsp olive or rapeseed oil**
* **1 clove garlic, crushed**
* **255g/9oz/1 heaping cup canned chopped tomatoes**
* **Pinch of thyme**
* **Pinch of oregano**
* **455g/1lb frozen mixed vegetables**
* **Salt and pepper**

1 Cook the pasta in lightly salted boiling water according to the instructions on the packet.
2 Meanwhile, heat the oil in a non-stick pan. Add the garlic and stir for a few seconds.
3 Pour in the tomatoes. Stir-fry until the tomatoes become soft and mushy (about 4–5 minutes).
4 Add the thyme, oregano, vegetables and seasoning. Cover and cook over a medium heat for about 5 minutes until the vegetables are cooked. Add a little hot water if the mixture begins to stick to the pan.
5 Mix in the drained, cooked pasta. Heat through and serve.

Healthy Eating Notes

Add a can of pulses like kidney beans or haricot beans to make this recipe a more substantial vegetarian meal.

Courgette and Mushroom Pizza

A crisp salad, ideally one with beans or sweetcorn, would make this into a delicious, nutritious meal.

Preparation time: 10 minutes
Cooking time: 10 minutes
Serves: 3

- 1 ready-made pizza base, roughly 25cm/10-inches in diameter
- A little olive oil, for brushing
- 2 tbsp tomato purée (paste)
- $^1/_2$ tsp dried oregano
- 1 courgette (zucchini), cut diagonally into thin slices
- 170g/6oz/2 cups mushrooms, sliced
- $^1/_2$ red (bell) pepper, cut into strips
- Salt and pepper
- 85g/3oz/$^3/_4$ cup reduced-fat Cheddar cheese, grated
- 1 tomato, sliced

1 Preheat the oven to 220°C/425°F/Gas Mark 7.
2 Brush the pizza bases with a little oil. Spread the tomato purée over the pizza base. Sprinkle the oregano on top.
3 Arrange the courgette (zucchini) slices, mushrooms and pepper strips over the pizza. Season with salt and pepper.
4 Add the cheese and decorate with the sliced tomato.
5 Place the pizza directly onto the oven shelf and cook for 15 minutes until the cheese is brown and bubbling.

Healthy Eating Notes

People with diabetes are encouraged to eat more starchy foods. Pizza is high in starchy carbohydrate. However, pizzas bought from fast-food outlets tend to be very high in fat as a lot of oil is used to make the base crisp and it is then smothered with full-fat mozzarella cheese. That's fine on occasions, but if you're a pizza-holic, then maybe experiment with this recipe, using different vegetable-based toppings.

Speedy Pizza Baguettes

Even the kids can get stuck in to this fun and easy recipe. A bread base makes a nice change from traditional pizza bases. Try this with some sweetcorn and a mixed salad.

Preparation time: 10 minutes
Cooking time: 5 minutes
Serves: 4

- **35cm/14-inch French baton loaf, cut into two and split lengthways**
- **A little olive oil, for brushing**
- **2 tbsp tomato purée (paste)**
- **$1/2$–1 tsp oregano, as desired**
- **55g/2oz/$1/2$ cup reduced-fat Cheddar cheese, grated**
- **2 tomatoes, sliced**
- **8 pitted olives, halved**

1 Preheat the grill (broiler) to medium.
2 Brush each piece of the cut side of the bread with olive oil.
3 Spread the tomato purée evenly over the bread. Sprinkle the oregano on top.
4 Cover this with a layer of cheese. Arrange the tomato slices and olives over the cheese.
5 Grill (broil) on a wire rack for about 3–5 minutes until the cheese has melted, and serve immediately.

Healthy Eating Notes

You can combine foods so that if you eat a lower-fibre dish, you can add salad or vegetables. This recipe uses white bread. Although wholemeal and granary varieties of bread are preferable because they are higher in fibre, and hence good for a healthy digestive system, you don't need to choose them all the time.

Bean, Pea and Sweetcorn Cottage Pie

This quick and easy dish is so veggie that, if it had more vegetables, it would still be in the ground! If you are really pushed for time, you could even make it with instant mash, although it's much nicer with fresh potatoes.

Preparation time: 10 minutes
Cooking time: 20 minutes
Serves: 4

- 565g/1¼lb/4 cups potatoes, peeled and diced
- 140g/5oz/1 cup frozen petits pois
- 200g/7oz/1 cup frozen sweetcorn
- Salt and white pepper
- 55g/2oz/½ cup low-fat cheddar cheese, grated
- 500g/18oz/2 cups canned baked beans in tomato sauce

1 Put the potatoes into boiling, salted water and cook for about 8 minutes until tender.
2 While the potatoes are cooking, cook the petits pois and sweetcorn in simmering water for about 4 minutes and drain well.
3 Drain the potatoes, mash well and season to taste with salt and pepper.
4 Mix in the cheddar cheese.
5 Add the baked beans to the peas and sweetcorn, reheat and transfer to a shallow gratin dish.
6 Top with the mashed potato, smooth the top and put under a hot grill (broiler) for about 5 minutes or until browned on top.
7 Serve piping hot.

Healthy Eating Notes

Frozen peas and sweetcorn take only minutes to cook and are just as high in vitamin C as fresh vegetables.

Greek Potatoes with Feta Cheese

This main-meal vegetarian choice only needs some fresh mixed salad as an accompaniment.

Preparation time: 15 minutes
Cooking time: 15–20 minutes
Serves: 4

- 900g/2lb potatoes, peeled and sliced thinly
- 4 spring onions (scallions), chopped
- 2 courgettes (zucchini) (about 225g/8oz), sliced thinly
- 85g/3oz feta cheese, cut into small cubes
- Freshly ground black pepper
- 1 tbsp Greek yoghurt
- 2 tbsp skimmed milk
- 1 tbsp olive oil

1 Preheat the oven to 375°F/190°C/Gas Mark 5. Lightly grease a large ovenproof dish.
2 Boil the potatoes in lightly salted water for 10 minutes.
3 Layer the potatoes, onions, courgettes (zucchini) and cheese into the dish, sprinkling some pepper in between.
4 Mix the yoghurt with the milk and pour over the vegetables.
5 Drizzle the oil over the top, cover the dish with foil and bake until the vegetables are cooked (about 20 minutes).

Healthy Eating Notes

Feta cheese has a salty flavour which enables you to use the minimum amount of salt when preparing the rest of the dish. It is important to cut down on salt because it is associated with high blood pressure.

Stuffed Peppers

The traditional recipe for stuffed peppers can take around 40 minutes in the oven as well as preparation time for the rice filling. This method takes a less conventional but easy short cut. The peppers cook in boiling water while you prepare the filling, so no time is wasted. The meal can be on the table in around half an hour. Use this recipe for leftovers too. Almost anything can be stuffed into the cooked peppers; they look appetizing and one pepper per person is sufficient for a light lunch or supper. Serve with a mixed salad or Red Cabbage Coleslaw (*see page 152*) and extra bread.

Preparation and cooking time: 30 minutes
Serves: 4

- **4 red (bell) peppers**
- **2 tsp corn oil**
- **1 onion, finely chopped**
- **2 cloves garlic, crushed**
- **115g/4oz frozen peas**
- **115g/4oz frozen sweetcorn**
- **1 tsp dried mixed herbs**
- **Salt and black pepper**
- **2 tbsp fresh parsley, chopped**
- **115g/4oz/$^1/_2$ cup long-grain rice, boiled**
- **30g/1oz/$^1/_4$ cup reduced-fat Cheddar cheese**

1 Cut a circle round the stem end of each pepper and remove the seeds. Put this circle back onto the peppers to form a lid. Place the peppers upright in a saucepan half-filled with boiling water. Bring back to the boil, cover and cook for 5 minutes.

2 Meanwhile, heat the oil in a non-stick pan. Add the onion and garlic and fry over a gentle heat to soften.

3 Add the peas, sweetcorn and seasoning to the pan with a few tablespoons of hot water. Cover with a tight-fitting lid and cook the vegetables over a high heat for a few minutes.

4 Add the parsley and rice to the vegetables and stir gently until well mixed.

5 Spoon the rice mixture into the peppers, sprinkle with grated cheese and cover with the 'lids'. Serve.

Healthy Eating Notes

Vegetable dishes combined with a starchy carbohydrate like rice or pasta are generally quick and easy to make and can be just as nourishing as meat-based meals.

Herb Mushrooms on Toast

Preparation and cooking time: 10 minutes
Serves: 3

- 1 tbsp olive oil
- 1 clove garlic, crushed
- 225g/8oz/2 cups mushrooms, sliced
- 2 tbsp fresh thyme or basil, finely chopped
- 2 tbsp fresh parsley, finely chopped
- Salt and coarsely ground black pepper
- 3 slices granary bread, toasted
- 1 tsp sesame seeds

1 Heat the oil in a non-stick frying pan (skillet) or wok. Add the garlic and mushrooms and stir-fry for a few minutes till the mushrooms are almost cooked.
2 Mix in the herbs and seasoning and cook for a further minute to soften the herbs.
3 Arrange the mushrooms on top of the toast and sprinkle with sesame seeds.

Healthy Eating Notes

A crunchy, low-calorie, low-fat, snappy supper dish or light vegetarian snack.

Curried Egg on Toast

A light snack consisting of spiced scrambled egg.

Preparation and cooking time: 10 minutes
Serves: 2

- **1 tsp rapeseed oil**
- **3 spring onions (scallions), sliced**
- **2 eggs, beaten**
- **1 green chilli, deseeded and finely chopped**
- **2 tbsp skimmed milk**
- **Pinch of turmeric**
- **Pinch of curry powder**
- **3 tbsp chopped coriander (cilantro) leaves**
- **Salt and pepper**
- **2 slices bread (preferably wholegrain), toasted, to serve**

1 Heat the oil in a non-stick frying pan (skillet). Add the onions and fry gently for 1 minute.
2 Mix the eggs with the chilli, milk, turmeric and curry powder.
3 Add the egg mix to the pan and stir gently till the egg is cooked.
4 Mix in the coriander (cilantro) and add the seasoning if necessary. Serve immediately on top of the toast.

Healthy Eating Notes

Eggs contain cholesterol, but the cholesterol in foods has very little effect on your blood cholesterol. This is because blood cholesterol is more influenced by the amount of saturated fat (such as full-fat dairy products and fatty meat) in your diet.

Spanish Omelette

This is a wonderful dish to make when you have odd bits of peppers and tomatoes in the fridge. It's also a good way of using up leftover boiled potatoes. Vary it by adding tuna or ham if you prefer a non-vegetarian option. You can serve it hot or cold – the Spanish way – with lots of toasted wholemeal or granary bread and a side salad.

Preparation and cooking time: 15 minutes
Serves: 3

- **3 eggs, beaten**
- **1 tbsp skimmed milk**
- **Salt and pepper**
- **1 small onion, finely chopped**
- **¼ green (bell) pepper, finely chopped**
- **1 tomato, chopped**
- **1 potato (about 140g/5oz), peeled, chopped and boiled**

1 Preheat the grill (broiler) to medium. Mix the eggs with the milk and seasoning.
2 Brush a non-stick frying pan (skillet) with a little oil. Heat the pan and add the onion and pepper. Fry for a few minutes to soften them.
3 Add the tomato, potato and the egg mixture. Stir for a few seconds and then allow the egg to set over a low heat for a few minutes.
4 Place the pan under the grill for two minutes until set and golden. Serve immediately.

Healthy Eating Notes

Eggs are a good source of protein and iron. Adding vegetables makes this into a more substantial and nutritious dish. Use a good non-stick frying pan (skillet) so you minimize the amount of oil needed in preparation.

Side dishes

Made the main part of the meal, got some pasta or potatoes on the boil, but still need a little something else? These accompaniments are designed to enhance the flavour of your dishes and to give you ideas on how to dress up vegetables when you want a change from steamed or boiled varieties. Choose dishes such as Hot Roasted Vegetables or Tomato and Coriander Salad to add colour, variety and essential nutrients.

Vegetables provide vitamins such as betacarotene (which appears in red, yellow and orange vegetables and is converted by the body to vitamin A) and vitamin C. Serving raw vegetables in salads or with dips is a great way of making sure you're getting enough of these nutrients. These 'antioxidant' vitamins are thought to protect against heart disease. Try to get into the habit of including at least one helping of vegetables or salad at every meal.

Bought salad dressings can add fat and calories to an otherwise healthy dish. In this chapter, you'll find ideas for salad dressings based on low-fat natural yoghurt and lemon juice. Alternatively, choose fat-free dressings from the supermarket.

Several of the recipes contain beans, sweetcorn or peas. These provide an important source of soluble fibre which helps to control your blood glucose level. Further, these vegetables are a cheap, low-fat source of protein.

Crisp Potato Rosti

Should you add onion to potato rosti? The Swiss don't, as a rule, but I think it gives the rosti a definite 'lift', so let's just say it's optional. You could even add some crumbled grilled crispy bacon, if you feel like it. Traditionally, raw potatoes are used in the recipe, but here they're parboiled for extra speed.

Preparation time: 10 minutes
Cooking time: 15–20 minutes
Serves: 4

- **680g/1¹/₂lb potatoes, peeled and halved**
- **30g/1oz/¹/₄ cup onion, grated**
- **1 tbsp plain (all purpose) flour**
- **1 egg, beaten**
- **15ml/1 tbsp sunflower oil**

1 Boil the potatoes in salted water for 10 minutes, turn into a colander and place under cold running water for a minute or so to make them cold enough to handle.
2 Grate them coarsely (or just mash them if you haven't the patience), then mix them together with the grated onion, flour and beaten egg.
3 Form into 4 large or 8 small cakes.
4 Heat the oil in a non-stick frying pan (skillet) and cook the potato cakes for 3–4 minutes on each side until crisp and golden.

Healthy Eating Notes

Potato rosti are often very oily, but cooking them with a small amount of oil in a non-stick pan helps to keep the fat down. Coarsely grated potato absorbs less fat than finely grated potato.

Southern Fries

If you love your chips but always thought they were too naughty to indulge in, here's a lower-fat way of having chips with extra flavour. Serve this dish with any meal you would normally like to have chips with. Reduce the amount of spices if you're cooking for young children who may prefer plainer flavours.

Preparation time: 5 minutes
Cooking time: 15 minutes
Serves: 2

- 200g/7oz 5 per cent fat oven chips
- 1 tsp Cajun seasoning
- 1/4 tsp dried mixed herbs
- 1/2 tsp dill pepper (optional)
- Pinch of salt

1 Preheat the grill (broiler) to medium. Line the grill pan with cooking foil.
2 Place the frozen chips in one layer on the grill pan.
3 Mix all the seasonings together.
4 Coat the chips with the seasoning and cook under the grill for 10–12 minutes, turning once during cooking.

Healthy Eating Notes

Chips bought from fish and chip shops can contain as much as 13 per cent fat. French fries sold in fast-food outlets have around 15 per cent fat. Choose reduced-fat oven chips instead.

Potato Wedges

Preparation time: 10 minutes

Cooking time: 15 minutes

Serves: 4

- 3 baking potatoes, washed and scrubbed
- 2 tbsp rapeseed or olive oil
- 2 tsp Chinese five-spice powder or dill pepper
- Salt and freshly ground black pepper

1 Preheat the grill (broiler) to high and line the grill pan with foil.
2 Cut each potato lengthways into 8 wedges. Boil in lightly salted water until just cooked. Drain.
3 Lightly grease the foil and put the cooked potatoes into the grill pan. Season with the five-spice powder and pepper.
4 Drizzle or brush the oil over the wedges and brown for 5–10 minutes under a hot grill. Serve immediately.

Healthy Eating Notes

Boiling, brushing with oil and grilling (broiling) potatoes can still produce crisp, golden potato wedges which taste every bit as good as the traditional deep-fried version – without the extra fat!

Creamed Potatoes with Cabbage

A delicious vegetable accompaniment to meat. The crunchy cabbage contrasts beautifully with the creamy texture of the potatoes. Serve in place of ordinary potatoes or rice.

Preparation and cooking time: 15 minutes
Serves: 4

- 125g/4^1/$_2$oz packet instant mashed potato mix
- 2 tbsp (40g) half-fat crème fraîche
- Salt and pepper
- 455g/1lb white cabbage, shredded and boiled
- 1 tbsp chopped fresh chives

1 Make up the mashed potato with boiling water according to the instructions on the packet. Blend in the half-fat crème fraîche and season.
2 Add the cabbage and chives and mix well.

Healthy Eating Notes

Mixing vegetables like cabbage with starchy foods such as potatoes is a great way of getting the kids to eat vegetables!

Cabbage with Fennel Seeds

If thinking of cabbage conjures up images of soggy cabbage at school dinners, then try this version which boasts lightly cooked white cabbage with the unusual taste of fennel seeds. This dish works well with grated carrots and shredded savoy cabbage too – use a combination of equal amounts of each.

Preparation and cooking time: 10 minutes
Serves: 4

- **455g/1lb white cabbage, sliced**
- **1 tbsp olive oil**
- **2 tsp fennel seeds**
- **Salt and coarsely ground black pepper**
- **Pinch cayenne pepper**

1 Steam the cabbage quickly until just cooked. Drain.
2 Heat the oil. Add the cabbage and stir-fry with the fennel seeds. Season, sprinkle on some cayenne pepper and serve.

Healthy Eating Notes

Including vegetable-based side dishes in a meal is a good way to increase your intake of nutrient-rich vegetables.

Red Cabbage Coleslaw

A filling portion size to complement any meal.

Preparation time: 15 minutes
Serves: 4

- 225g/8oz/4 cups red cabbage, shredded or grated
- 3 carrots, grated
- 3 spring onions (scallions), sliced
- 115ml/4fl oz/$^1/_2$ cup reduced-calorie mayonnaise

1 Simply mix all the ingredients together and serve!

Healthy Eating Notes

The reduced-calorie mayonnaise helps to keep the fat lower than standard coleslaw. If you want to get it down further, choose a low-fat natural yoghurt or fat-free vinaigrette instead.

Creamy Carrot and Parsnip Purée

This makes a delicious accompaniment to roast beef, but would also go well with any winter stew (great with Pork Steaks with Creamy Mustard Sauce, *page 52*). The big advantage is that the two vegetables are cooked together, so that's one less pan to wash up! For a variation, try using yellow turnip instead of parsnips.

Preparation time: 5 minutes
Cooking time: 15 minutes
Serves: 4

- **285g/10oz/2 cups carrots, coarsely diced**
- **285g/10oz/2 cups parsnips, coarsely diced**
- **1 tbsp low-fat spread**
- **Salt and pepper to taste**
- **Sprinkling freshly chopped parsley**

1 Put the vegetables into a pan of salted water and bring to the boil. Lower the heat and cook for 8–10 minutes till tender.
2 Drain, mash and beat in the low-fat spread.
3 Season to taste and serve garnished with freshly chopped parsley.

Healthy Eating Notes

Carrots are a rich source of betacarotene. The body converts this to vitamin A, which has beneficial, antioxidant properties that protect against heart disease.

Minted Carrot Salad

Preparation time: 10 minutes

Serves: 4

- **4 carrots, diced**
- **1 tsp mint sauce**
- **55g/2oz/¹/₂ cup raisins**

1 Simply mix and serve.

Healthy Eating Notes

Although dried fruits are high in sugar, it is perfectly acceptable to use them if you have diabetes.

Tomato and Coriander Salad

A refreshing accompaniment to any meal.

Preparation time: 10 minutes
Serves: 4

- **455g/1lb/2¹/₂ cups tomatoes, thinly sliced**
- **4 spring onions (scallions), finely sliced**
- **15g/¹/₂ oz packet fresh coriander (cilantro), chopped**
- **Coarsely ground black pepper**
- **Lemon juice, to taste**

1 Simply mix all the ingredients together and serve.

Healthy Eating Notes

Tomatoes are rich in betacarotene which is converted into vitamin A in the body. Vegetables, especially raw vegetables, are also good sources of vitamin C. Vitamins A, C and E are antioxidant vitamins which are thought to help in the prevention of heart disease.

Five-Minute Potato Salad

Preparation time: 5 minutes

Serves: 4

- **540g/19oz can unpeeled potatoes, drained**
- **140ml/5fl oz/²/₃ cup low-fat natural yoghurt**
- **3 tbsp fresh chives, snipped**
- **Salt and coarse black pepper**

1 Cut the potatoes into halves.
2 Mix the yoghurt with the chives and seasoning.
3 Dress the potatoes with the yoghurt mixture and serve chilled.

Healthy Eating Notes

Unpeeled potatoes help to provide fibre, and low-fat yoghurt makes an excellent substitute for full-fat, or even reduced-calorie, mayonnaise.

Hot Beetroot and Apple with Creamy Horseradish

This is just what you need to give a lift to the rather mundane grilled pork chop, and it's even better if pork is on the menu for the Sunday roast. Raw beetroot can sometimes be hard to find and takes more preparation, so cut corners and buy it ready-cooked (but not in vinegar).

Preparation time: 10 minutes
Cooking time: 10 minutes
Serves: 4

- **455g/1lb dessert apples, peeled, cored and sliced**
- **255g/9oz/1^1/$_2$ cups cooked beetroot, diced**
- **10ml/2 tsp hot horseradish sauce**
- **30ml/2 tbsp lower-fat Greek yoghurt**
- **Freshly ground black pepper**

1 Put the apples into a pan with a little water (30ml/2 tbsp should be enough), and bring to the boil.
2 Lower the heat and simmer for about 8 minutes or until soft and pulpy.
3 Stir in the diced beetroot.
4 Mix the horseradish sauce with the yoghurt and stir into the mixture.
5 Reheat for a minute or so, then season to taste with black pepper before serving.

Healthy Eating Notes

The apples and beetroot in this recipe count towards your daily intake of fruit and vegetables.

Stir-fried Baby Corn and Mangetout

This colourful recipe is packed with flavour and the crunchy peanuts add an exciting texture.

Preparation time: 5 minutes
Cooking time: 5–8 minutes
Serves: 4

- **200g/7oz baby corn**
- **5ml/1 tsp sesame oil**
- **170g/6oz mangetout**
- **140g/5oz spring onions (scallions), roots removed and chopped diagonally (approx. 2cm/³/₄-inch long)**
- **40g/1¹/₂oz peanuts, chopped**

1 Part-cook the baby corn by heating in the microwave in water for 3 minutes on high (or simmer for the same time in a saucepan).
2 Drain and then cut each corncob in half.
3 Heat a wok to a high temperature then add the sesame oil.
4 Add the mangetout, spring onions and baby corn pieces and continue to stir-fry on high for 3 minutes.
5 Sprinkle with the nuts, mix and serve.

Healthy Eating Notes

Peanuts are certainly high in fat, but did you know that they have a low glycaemic index? So, in diabetes, they may actually help keep your blood glucose levels steady. Sprinkle them into foods in this way to add valuable nutrients – a handful a day is perfectly acceptable as part of a healthy diet, but be careful how much you eat if you are trying to lose weight.

Curried Sweetcorn

Although this is a side dish, I must confess to having half the recipe as a main meal, served with low-fat natural yoghurt and lots of naan bread – can you resist it? A yummy meal or snack that's on the table in 10 minutes. This side dish has quite a strong flavour, so use it to spice up an otherwise bland meal. It can be served on toast, or with any main dish and fresh salad.

Preparation and cooking time: 10 minutes
Serves: 4

- **2 tsp corn oil**
- **1 tsp cumin seeds**
- **1 tbsp tomato purée (paste)**
- **2 tsp curry powder**
- **325g/11½oz can sweetcorn**
- **2 spring onions (scallions), sliced**
- **2 tbsp fresh coriander (cilantro), chopped**

1 Heat the oil in a non-stick pan. Add the cumin seeds and let them pop for only a few seconds.
2 Stir in the tomato purée and curry powder, and blend together well over a low heat.
3 Mix in the sweetcorn, spring onions (scallions) and coriander (cilantro). Add a few tablespoons of hot water if you prefer more sauce, and serve hot.

Healthy Eating Notes

Vegetables are high in soluble fibre which helps you to control blood glucose levels more easily. This type of fibre has also been shown to lower blood fats such as cholesterol. Try to eat two large helpings of vegetables per day.

Creamy Broad Beans

A scrumptious way to serve up an otherwise bland vegetable. This fibre-rich dish can complement an otherwise low-fibre main course.

Preparation and cooking time: 10 minutes
Serves: 2

- **200g/7oz/1 cup frozen broad beans**
- **55g/2oz medium-fat soft cheese**
- **$1/_4$ tsp dried mixed herbs**
- **Salt and coarsely ground black pepper**

1 Cook the beans in lightly salted boiling water in a covered pan. This should take 4–5 minutes.
2 Meanwhile, mix the cheese with the seasonings.
3 Stir the flavoured cheese into the drained beans, adjust the seasoning and heat through.

Healthy Eating Notes

Try to eat two large helpings of vegetables per day. Vegetables are good sources of the antioxidant vitamins A and C. Antioxidants are thought to protect against heart disease.

Sesame Green Beans

Tired of plain boiled vegetables? Make an interesting change with this recipe which you can use with any vegetables of your choice.

Preparation and cooking time: 10 minutes
Serves: 4

- **455g/1lb/5 cups frozen French beans**
- **1 tsp olive oil**
- **2 tbsp sesame seeds**

1 Boil the beans quickly till just cooked.
2 Heat the oil. Add the sesame seeds and then the drained, cooked beans. Stir till the beans are well coated with the seeds.

Healthy Eating Notes

Cook vegetables lightly in a minimum of water over a high heat to help preserve the vitamin C. Serving them immediately after cooking also helps to maintain the vitamin C content.

Barbecue Baked Beans

Baked beans are an excellent convenience food. This recipe adds variety to standard baked beans in a matter of minutes. A delicious accompaniment to any meal, or serve on granary toast or in jacket potatoes.

Preparation and cooking time: 5 minutes
Serves: 2

- **425g/15oz can baked beans in tomato sauce**
- **1 tbsp Worcester sauce**
- **1 tbsp vinegar**
- **1 tbsp soy sauce**
- **Coarsely ground black pepper**
- **Pinch of mustard powder (optional)**

1 Simply add all the ingredients to the beans in a pan, heat and serve.

Healthy Eating Notes

Baked beans are made from haricot beans, which are a pulse vegetable. Pulses are high in soluble fibre. This type of fibre is slowly absorbed by the body, so it helps to minimize 'highs' and 'lows' in blood glucose.

Three Bean Salad

This fibre-rich side dish is a gre‌͏ ͏‌nt to a low-fibre meal.
Serve it with quiches and piz‍ ‍‍ith a jacket potato filled with
cottage cheese.

Preparation time: 1͏
Serves·

- 425g/‍ ͏kpeas, drained
- **425g/15o͏‌ ͏idney beans, drained**
- **425g/15oz can blackeye beans, drained**
- **3 spring onions (scallions), chopped**
- **2 tbsp chopped parsley**

For the dressing
- **4 tbsp low-fat natural yoghurt**
- **2 tbsp cider vinegar**
- **2 tbsp olive oil**
- **Salt and pepper**

1 Add the chickpeas and beans to the spring onions and parsley in a large salad bowl.
2 Put the dressing ingredients into a screw-top jar, cover with a tight-fitting lid and shake well.
3 Pour the dressing over the beans. Chill in the refrigerator and stir just before serving.

Healthy Eating Notes

The low-fat yoghurt dressing adds flavour without the calories of traditional salad dressings.

Peas with Shallots

Preparation time: 5 minutes
Cooking time: 5 minutes
Serves: 4

- 1 vegetable stock cube, made up to 140ml/¼ pint/⅔ cup with boiling water
- 340g/12oz/2½ cups frozen peas
- 8 button onions or shallots, peeled and halved
- Good pinch of marjoram
- Salt and pepper

1 Put all the ingredients into a pan with a tight-fitting lid.
2 Bring back to the boil. Cover and simmer till the peas are cooked and the onions are softened.

Healthy Eating Notes

Try to have two large helpings of vegetables daily, and choose peas, beans or lentils often as they are a good source of soluble fibre.

Hot Roasted Vegetables

This recipe combines traditional root vegetables, such as carrots, parsnips and swedes (rutabaga), and gives them a more Mediterranean flavour.

Preparation time: 20 minutes
Cooking time: 15 minutes
Serves: 4

- **455g/1lb/3^1/$_4$ cups carrots, cut into matchsticks**
- **455g/1lb/3^1/$_4$ cups parsnips, cut into matchsticks**
- **455g/1lb/3^1/$_4$ cups swedes or turnips (rutabaga), diced**
- **2 tsp olive oil**
- **2 tbsp pine nuts**
- **1 clove garlic, crushed**
- **Pinch of dried herbs**
- **2 tbsp chopped parsley**
- **Salt and pepper**

1 Preheat the oven to 375°F/190°C/Gas Mark 5. Lightly grease an ovenproof dish.
2 Cook the vegetables for 3–4 minutes in boiling water.
3 Drain the vegetables and mix with the other ingredients.
4 Put the mixture into the dish and roast in the oven for about 15 minutes.

Healthy Eating Notes

People in the UK eat less fruit and vegetables than is recommended for good health. Try to eat five portions of fruit and vegetables (not counting potatoes) a day. Vegetables are low in calories, high in fibre and most are fat-free. Preparing dishes such as this makes a refreshing change from boiled vegetables.

Salsa Sauce

Add a touch of Mexico to your meals with this crunchy, lightly spiced sauce. Serve hot or cold as a relish for hamburgers or lean grilled chops.

Preparation and cooking time: 15 minutes
Serves: 4

- **1 tsp corn oil**
- **1 clove garlic, crushed**
- **1 small onion, finely chopped**
- **$1/_2$ green (bell) pepper, diced**
- **200g/7oz/1 scant cup canned chopped tomatoes in tomato juice**
- **$1/_4$ tsp red chilli powder**

1 Heat the oil in a non-stick frying pan (skillet).
2 Add the garlic, onion and pepper, and fry gently for about 4–5 minutes.
3 Add the tomatoes and chilli. Lower the heat and simmer for about 5 minutes, stirring occasionally.

Healthy Eating Notes
Canned tomatoes are packed with the antioxidant lycopene, so don't feel you always have to use fresh ones to get the benefits.

Cucumber and Mint Raita

Preparation time: 10 minutes

Serves: 4

- 500g/18oz carton low-fat natural yoghurt
- 1 tbsp chopped fresh mint
- $1/2$ tsp coarsely ground black pepper
- $1/2$ cucumber, grated

1 Season the yoghurt with the mint and pepper. Chill.
2 Just before serving, stir in the cucumber.

Healthy Eating Notes

Choose low-fat dairy products (such as low-fat yoghurt, low-fat fromage frais, reduced-calorie mayonnaise) wherever possible. Low-fat dairy foods can help you to cut down on your saturated fat intake so long as you don't eat more of them than the full-fat version.

Instant Mint Chutney

A runny chutney which is great when used as a dipping sauce for chicken drumsticks or sausages (lower-fat ones, of course!). If you prefer a thicker chutney, simply add less water.

Preparation time: 5 minutes
Serves: 3

- **2 tbsp tomato ketchup**
- **1 tsp mint sauce**
- **$1/4$–$1/2$ tsp red chilli powder**
- **2 tbsp cold water**

1 Simply mix all the ingredients together!

Crunchy Cucumber Relish

Preparation time: 10 minutes

Serves: 4

- **1 cucumber, diced**
- **40g/1¹/₂oz chopped nuts, e.g. peanuts**
- **1 tbsp lemon juice**
- **Salt and coarsely ground black pepper**

1 Simply mix and serve.

Healthy Eating Notes

Nuts and seeds are a good source of vitamins and minerals, especially vitamin E and zinc. These are needed in small amounts for good health.

Desserts

Banana and Chocolate Pie and Pears in Blackcurrant Sauce are only a couple of the tempting treats you'll find in this chapter. Having diabetes doesn't mean saying goodbye to those sweet endings to your meals. All sorts of desserts can be incorporated into a healthy diet, particularly if you choose appropriate ingredients. Half-fat creams, low-fat instant dessert mixes and fresh fruit have been suggested in these recipes as they help to reduce the fat and sugar content of traditional puds. To cut down even further on fat, try using virtually fat-free fromage frais or low-fat natural yoghurt.

Base desserts on fresh fruit as often as possible and try to eat three pieces of fruit every day.

Pan-fried Bananas with Sticky Toffee Crumble

Yes, they've got sugar; yes, they've got butter – but really very little of each, and the taste is just heaven from a pan! They are also very filling, so have them after something light. If you like, you can use wholemeal breadcrumbs, but ready-bought white ones give a nicer, more golden colour when cooked. If you can't find them, make your own from the equivalent weight in slightly stale bread. Cut off the crusts and whiz in a blender or food processor for a few seconds.

Preparation time: 5 minutes
Cooking time: 10 minutes
Serves: 4

- 30g/1oz butter
- 30g/1oz/2 tbsp demerara sugar
- 4 x 170g/6oz bananas, peeled and halved lengthways
- 45g/1^1/$_2$oz/^{3}/$_4$ cup white breadcrumbs
- 45ml/3 tbsp low-fat Greek yoghurt

1 Melt the butter gently in a large, non-stick frying pan (skillet), taking care not to let it brown.
2 Add the sugar and cook very gently for 2–3 minutes until dissolved.
3 Add the bananas, cut-side down, and cook for a further 2–3 minutes, using 2 wooden spoons to turn them over. (Don't worry if they break up – they'll still taste the same!)
4 Add the breadcrumbs and stir-cook, raising the heat a little, until brown and crisp.
5 Serve while still warm and sticky, with the chilled Greek yoghurt.

Healthy Eating Notes

The bananas count towards your recommended daily intake of fruit. Low-fat yoghurt helps keep the fat content down.

Banana and Chocolate Pie

No rolling of pastry, no baking. All you need is a knife and a whisk and you can create this scrumptious dessert in 15 minutes.

This recipe is far lower in fat than standard creamy pies, but to keep an eye on your fat intake, serve it after a low-fat main course, such as Vegetable Pasta in Tomato Sauce (*see page 135*), which has less than 5 per cent fat.

Preparation time: 15 minutes
Serves: 8

- 49g/1³/₄oz packet sugar-free chocolate-flavour whipped dessert mix, e.g. Angel Delight
- 285ml/¹/₂ pint/1¹/₃ cups skimmed milk
- 3 bananas, sliced or mashed
- 18cm/7-inch bought pastry case
- 90ml/3fl oz/¹/₃ cup half-fat whipping cream
- ¹/₂ bar chocolate flake, crumbled
- 20g/³/₄oz chopped nuts

1 Make up the whipped dessert with the skimmed milk according to the instructions on the packet.
2 Put the bananas into the pastry case. Cover with the made-up dessert.
3 Whip the cream and layer on top.
4 Sprinkle the chocolate crumbs and nuts over the cream. Chill and serve.

Healthy Eating Notes

Although the bought pastry case is just as high in fat and sugar as ordinary sweet pastry, this recipe uses sugar-free mousse for the filling and half-fat cream for the topping. This makes it lower in fat than standard creamy pies.

Hot Bananas with Almonds

A naturally sweet, easy dessert that takes just over five minutes to prepare. The bananas are split, flavoured with almonds and raisins and then sandwiched together. They are cooked in their own skin, so all the juices are preserved. This is a great way to prepare bananas if you are planning a barbecue, as they can be cooked on the charcoal in their skins. Since each banana is served wrapped in its parcel of foil, it's also a fun and sneaky way to get kids to eat fruit!

Preparation time: 5–10 minutes
Cooking time: 20 minutes
Serves: 4

- **4 bananas**
- **2 tbsp lemon juice**
- **30g/1oz flaked almonds**
- **30g/1oz raisins**

1 Preheat the oven to 220°C/425°F/Gas Mark 7.
2 Make one lengthways slit in each banana, keeping the skin as intact as possible. Sprinkle on the lemon juice.
3 Stuff the almonds and raisins into each banana.
4 Cover the whole banana with foil.
5 Repeat this with all the bananas. Place them directly onto the rack in the oven. Cook for 20–25 minutes till they are soft.

Healthy Eating Notes

People in the UK eat far less fruit than is recommended for health. Try to eat three pieces of fruit per day. Fruit is high in the antioxidant vitamins (A and C), which have been shown to be protective against heart disease.

Hot Chocolate and Chestnut Soufflés

If Eve had spotted these mini-soufflés, I doubt she'd have bothered with the apple, for they are almost sinfully indulgent, but oh-so-delicious! They have to be served in the little pots in which they are cooked, otherwise they will collapse, but there's no reason why you shouldn't go the whole hog on a special occasion and have a scoop of reduced-fat ice cream on the side.

Preparation time: 10 minutes
Cooking time: 15–20 minutes
Serves: 4

- **55g/2oz dark Swiss chocolate (70% cocoa)**
- **115g/4oz unsweetened chestnut purée**
- **1 tbsp caster (confectioner's) sugar**
- **1 egg yolk**
- **2 egg whites, stiffly beaten**
- **1 tsp butter or margarine to grease 4 ramekins**

1 Preheat the oven to 200°C/400°F/Gas Mark 6.
2 Break the chocolate into chunks, put in a small pan with 15ml/1 tbsp water and heat very gently until the chocolate has completely melted.
3 Add the chestnut purée and caster sugar and cook, stirring, until the sugar has dissolved.
4 Remove from the heat and stir in the egg yolk, mixing thoroughly.
5 Fold in the stiffly beaten egg whites, using a large metal spoon, and transfer the mixture to 4 lightly greased ramekins.
6 Stand the ramekins in a roasting tin with enough hot water to come halfway up their sides, and bake in the centre of the oven for 15–20 minutes until risen and set.

Healthy Eating Notes

This recipe does contain a fair amount of saturated fat, so perhaps save it for special occasions.

Baked Rice Darioles with Crushed Summer Berries

These little soufflés can be made in ramekins, dariole moulds or other small individual ovenproof dishes. They cook very quickly, because they use flaked rice, which cooks in just 5 or 6 minutes. The texture is much smoother than when made with traditional pudding rice, but they are still delicious, and you can of course use canned or frozen berries, provided they have no added sugar in the syrup.

Preparation time: 5 minutes
Cooking time: 25 minutes
Serves: 4

- **30g/1oz/2 tbsp flaked rice**
- **285ml/^{1}/$_2$ pint/1^1/$_3$ cups skimmed or semi-skimmed milk**
- **1 tbsp caster (confectioner's) sugar**
- **2–3 drops almond essence**
- **1 egg yolk**
- **2 egg whites, stiffly beaten**
- **1 tsp butter or margarine (to grease 4 ramekins)**
- **170g/6oz soft summer berries (raspberries, strawberries, blackcurrants or a mixture), drained if canned**

1 Preheat the oven to 200°C, 400°F, Gas Mark 6.
2 Put the rice into a small pan with the milk and caster sugar and bring gently to the boil, stirring to dissolve the sugar.
3 Cook for 5 minutes, stirring regularly, till thickened.
4 Remove from the heat, stir in the almond essence and egg yolk and mix thoroughly.
5 Lightly fold in the egg whites, using a large metal spoon, and divide the mixture among 4 lightly greased ramekins.
6 Stand the ramekins in a roasting tin filled with enough hot water to come halfway up their sides, and bake in the centre of the oven for 15–20 minutes until risen and set.

7 While they are baking, gently heat and crush the summer berries.

8 Serve the soufflés immediately, surrounded by the crushed berries.

Healthy Eating Notes

Summer berries are a rich source of vitamin C.

Grilled Pineapple Meringues

When using canned pineapple slices you may wish to double up the rings to make them thicker, but if using fresh pineapple, cut the slices to a thickness of about 2cm/1 inch instead. The meringue can be piped for a more professional finish and decorated with toasted almonds if desired.

Other fruits could also be used, such as peaches or fresh pears, or you could try mini-meringues with apricot halves.

Preparation time: 5 minutes
Cooking time: 5 minutes
Serves: 4

- **1 large egg white**
- **55g/2oz/¼ cup caster (confectioner's) sugar**
- **Pinch cornflour (cornstarch)**
- **1 can (425g/15oz/2 cups) pineapple slices in natural juice, drained**

1 Preheat the grill (broiler) to high.
2 Make the meringue by whisking the egg white in a dry bowl until soft peaks are formed.
3 Add the sugar mixed with the cornflour and continue whisking until well blended.
4 Place the drained pineapple rings on a grill tray and cook for 2 minutes, turning once.
5 Spoon meringue mixture on top of each pineapple slice and put back under the grill.
6 Cook for approximately 1–2 minutes until the meringue is golden, then serve.

Healthy Eating Notes

Although meringue is made from eggs, it is naturally low in fat as you use only the egg white.

Pineapple Muesli Crumble

No chopping of fruit, no tedious preparation of crumble toppings. Ready-made ingredients help you to prepare this hot pud in a jiffy. You can use a variety of accompaniments, depending on the occasion. Low-fat yoghurt, low-fat custard made up from a sachet and ice cream are much lower in fat than fresh cream. You could also try a spoonful of fromage frais or Greek yoghurt. The fruit in this recipe provides ample sweetness for the dish, so there is no need to use muesli with added sugar, whether or not you have diabetes.

Preparation time: 10 minutes
Cooking time: 25 minutes
Serves: 6

- **2 large bananas, sliced**
- **425g/15oz can crushed pineapple in pineapple juice**
- **140g/5oz sugar-free muesli**
- **1 tbsp corn oil**

1 Preheat the oven to 180°C/350°F/Gas Mark 4. Lightly grease an ovenproof dish.
2 Put the bananas, pineapple and juice into the bottom of the dish.
3 Mix the muesli with the oil. Pour this mixture over the fruit.
4 Cover with foil and bake in the centre of the oven for 20 minutes. Remove the foil and cook for a further 5 minutes.

Healthy Eating Notes

Muesli contains dried fruit, oats and nuts. Oats are particularly beneficial in diabetes because they contain soluble fibre which helps to slow down the rise in blood glucose after meals.

Mini Cherry Sponges

This is a classic cheat – using shop-bought plain sponge cake or little fairy cakes. The fairy cakes make an attractive change from a flat base.

Preparation time: 5 minutes
Cooking time: 5 minutes
Serves: 4

- **1 can (425g/15oz /2 cups) pitted black cherries in natural juice**
- **2 tsp arrowroot**

To serve
- **225g/8oz sponge fairy cakes**
- **4 tbsp low-fat natural yoghurt**

1 Drain the cherries from the juice and set them aside, reserving the juice.
2 Put the juice in a non-stick saucepan and add the arrowroot.
3 Heat until the juice thickens, stirring continuously, and return the cherries to the mixture, allowing them to warm.
4 Place the sponge cakes on the serving plate and pour over the cherry mixture.
5 Top with natural yoghurt and serve.

Healthy Eating Notes

Cherries count towards your daily intake of fruit, and the low-fat yoghurt helps keep the fat content down.

Yoghurt with Peach Sauce

A refreshing and light summer pudding. This peach sauce is so versatile you could serve it hot over a fruity crumble or as a fruit coulis with a fruit tart.

Preparation time: 5 minutes
Cooking time: 5 minutes
Chilling time: 20 minutes
Serves: 4

For the peach sauce
- **2 cans (395g/14oz/1 cup each) peaches tinned in natural juice, drained and puréed**
- **45g/3 tbsp reduced-sugar peach jam**

To serve
- **600ml/21fl oz/2¹/₂ cups low-fat natural yoghurt**

1 Take the puréed peaches and place in a saucepan with the jam.
2 Simmer for 5 minutes and then chill thoroughly.
3 Serve, swirled into low-fat natural yoghurt.

Healthy Eating Notes

This recipe is bursting with vitamin C. Low-fat yoghurt helps keep the fat content down.

Red Fruit Compote

Red fruit compote is an interesting variation on a traditional fruit salad. If desired, you could use a tablespoon of Cointreau instead of the wine or leave the alcohol out and use fresh orange juice instead.

Preparation time: 5 minutes
Chilling time: 20 minutes (more if desired)
Serves: 6

- 255g/9oz/1$\frac{1}{2}$ cups strawberries, hulled and cut into bite-sized pieces
- 140g/5oz/1 cup cherries, stoned
- 140g/5oz/1 cup raspberries
- 140g/5oz/1 cup blackberries
- 60ml/2fl oz/$\frac{1}{4}$ cup dry white wine, sparkling if possible
- 30g/1oz/2 tbsp icing (powdered) sugar
- Fresh mint sprigs

1 Wash all the fruit and make sure it has been cut into bite-sized pieces.
2 Place in a large serving bowl and pour over the wine.
3 Sprinkle with icing sugar and leave in a cold place to chill.
4 Mix once before serving and decorate with fresh mint.

Healthy Eating Notes

The fruits are a rich source of fibre and vitamin C. Choosing different fruits helps you get a variety of nutrients.

Home-made Waffles

Waffles are quick and easy to make and very versatile, but you do need a waffle iron. Alternatively, buy ready-made waffles and heat them up in the oven. Toppings such as Red Fruit Compote (*page 183*) or peach sauce (*page 184*) are scrumptious or you could simply top with some sliced banana and a dusting of icing (powdered) sugar.

Preparation time: 10 minutes
Cooking time: 10 minutes
Serves: 4

- **125g/4^1/$_2$oz /1 cup wholewheat plain (all purpose) flour**
- **2 tsp baking powder**
- **Pinch of salt**
- **1 egg**
- **15ml/1 tbsp sunflower oil**
- **170ml/6fl oz/^{2}/$_3$ cup skimmed milk**
- **15g/1 tbsp caster (confectioner's) sugar**

1 In a large bowl, mix together the flour, baking powder and salt.
2 Separate the egg and mix the yolk with the oil and the milk.
3 Add this to the dry ingredients and mix well into a batter.
4 Whisk the egg white until stiff, then add the sugar and mix again.
5 Fold the egg white and sugar into the batter.
6 Heat your waffle iron and add 3 tbsp of batter for each waffle.
7 Cook each waffle for 2–3 minutes and serve immediately.

Healthy Eating Notes

Waffles are a useful base for healthy fruit toppings and a good way to get kids to eat fruit.

Chocolate Pancakes with Orange

Chocolate and orange are a divine combination and this recipe is even better than the traditional lemon version of crêpes suzettes.

Preparation time: 10 minutes
Cooking time: 20 minutes
Serves: 4

- 115g/4oz/^{2}/$_3$ cup plain (all purpose) wholewheat flour
- 10g/2 tsp cocoa powder
- Pinch of salt
- 5ml/1 tsp vanilla extract
- 1 large orange, rind removed, peeled and segmented
- 100ml/3^1/$_2$fl oz/^{1}/$_2$ cup skimmed milk
- 2 eggs, beaten
- 10ml/2 tsp sunflower oil or a few sprays of spray oil
- 140ml/5fl oz /^{2}/$_3$ cup fresh unsweetened orange juice
- 10g/2 tsp caster (confectioner's) sugar (to garnish)

1 First, make the pancake batter. Mix the flour, cocoa powder, salt, vanilla extract and orange rind together in a large bowl.
2 Add the milk, then beat in the eggs.
3 Spray or drizzle a little sunflower oil onto a small pancake pan, heat to a high temperature and add ^{1}/$_8$ of the batter mixture.
4 Tilt it to spread the batter mixture and cook until the small bubbles in the mixture have started to burst.
5 Flip the pancake and cook for another 30 seconds to ensure the second side is cooked.
6 Place in foil to keep warm while you make the rest of the pancakes.
7 In a large frying pan (skillet), heat the orange juice.
8 Fold the pancakes into triangles and place in the orange juice to heat up.

9 Serve the pancakes with the orange segments and any remaining orange juice poured over.

10 Sprinkle with a dusting of caster sugar to decorate.

Healthy Eating Notes

By using wholewheat flour, you can boost your fibre intake for a healthy digestion.

Chinese Pears with Ginger

These look quite impressive for a dinner party if you leave the stalks on the pears. This also means they can be used as handles to remove the lids. Delicious served with reduced-fat fromage frais or yoghurt.

Preparation time: 10 minutes

Cooking time: 20 minutes

Serves: 4

- 55g/2oz/$^1/_3$ cup golden sultanas, chopped
- 55g/2oz/$^1/_3$ cup pine kernels, chopped
- 15ml/1 tbsp clear honey
- 15g/$^1/_2$oz /2 pieces crystallized ginger, chopped
- 4 ripe pears (Williams or broad shaped)
- 30g/1oz/2 tbsp reduced-sugar redcurrant jelly

1 Preheat the oven to 190°C/375°F/Gas Mark 5.
2 Mix the chopped sultanas and pine kernels with the honey and 1 piece of chopped ginger.
3 Prepare the pears by cutting approximately 2cm/1 inch off the top (leave the stalks attached).
4 Carefully scoop out the core and pips and then peel.
5 Stand them upright (so they have a level base) in an ovenproof dish.
6 Spoon the mixture into the core of the pears.
7 Peel the tops, then replace them on each pear (still with stalks attached).
8 Mix the redcurrant jelly with 25ml/5 tsp hot water and the remainder of the ginger.
9 Pour the liquid over the pears.
10 Cover and bake for 20 minutes.

Healthy Eating Notes

The pears and sultanas count towards your daily intake of fruit.

Gooseberry Fool

If you have the luxury of fresh gooseberries, stew them and use instead of the canned variety. Rhubarb is another fruit that goes particularly well in this recipe.

Preparation time: 5 minutes
Cooking time: 5 minutes
Chilling time: 20 minutes
Serves: 4

- **2 cans (285g/10oz/2 cups) gooseberries in natural juice, drained**
- **15g/1 tbsp custard powder**
- **15g/1 tbsp granulated sugar**
- **425ml/15fl oz/2 cups skimmed milk**
- **40g/1¹/₂oz/¹/₂ cup toasted, flaked almonds**
- **1 tbsp toasted almond flakes (to garnish)**
- **60ml/4 tbsp reduced-fat fromage frais (to garnish)**

1 Liquidize the gooseberries to a purée.
2 In a bowl, mix together the custard powder, sugar and 60ml/2fl oz/¹/₄ cup milk.
3 Heat the remaining milk in a saucepan until warm.
4 Add to the custard powder mixture, stir and return to the pan.
5 Stir over a medium heat until the custard thickens.
6 Remove from the heat, add the gooseberry purée and almonds and mix.
7 Pour into serving dishes and chill.
8 Decorate and serve.

Healthy Eating Notes
Fruit-based recipes, like this one, are a healthy option.

Apple Slices on Cinnamon Toast

Brioche is a luscious French bun made with a yeast dough. The apple and cinnamon complement the rich taste wonderfully. Serve with some natural yoghurt or half-fat crème fraîche.

Preparation and cooking time: 10 minutes
Serves: 4

- **2 eating apples (approx. 170g/6oz/1$\frac{1}{2}$ cups each)**
- **Juice of 1 lemon**
- **15g/1 tbsp caster (confectioner's) sugar**
- **$^1\!/_2$ tsp cinnamon**
- **115g/4oz brioche (preferably sliced from a loaf, but individual rolls would be fine)**

1 Preheat the grill (broiler) to high.
2 Peel and core the apples and cut each into 4 thick slices.
3 Sprinkle with lemon juice to prevent them browning.
4 Mix together the sugar and cinnamon.
5 Cut the brioche into 4 slices (if using a loaf) or cut the individual rolls in half and place on a grill tray. Place the apple slices alongside.
6 Grill the apple slices and brioche until the brioche is golden on one side.
7 Turn the brioche over and sprinkle with half of the sugar mixture.
8 Place the grilled apples on top and sprinkle with the remaining mixture.
9 Grill until brown and serve immediately.

Healthy Eating Notes

The apples count towards your daily intake of fruit.

Melon and Raspberry with Mint

Impress any guests by using a melon baller and serving in a melon shell. For extra wow factor, mix a variety of melon types such as pink watermelon, pale honeydew and bright-orange cantaloupe.

Preparation time: 10 minutes
Serves: 4

- 1 Galia melon (approx. 980g /35oz)
- 255g/9oz/2 cups fresh raspberries, washed and hulled
- 3 sprigs fresh mint, bruised (plus 8 mint leaves to garnish)
- 200ml/7fl oz/³/₄ cup dry white wine, chilled

1 Cut the melon into bite-sized pieces and discard the skin.
2 Put in a bowl with the raspberries and bruised mint sprigs.
3 Pour over the chilled wine and chill further for 5 minutes.
4 Remove the bruised mint and serve in individual glass dishes, garnished with mint leaves.

Healthy Eating Notes

This recipe is packed with fruit, making it a nutritious, low-fat option.

Biscuit and Strawberry Pudding

This dessert is high in fat, so save it for special occasions.

Preparation time: 20 minutes
Serves: 6

- **140g/5oz semi-sweet biscuits (e.g. Marie, Rich Tea), crushed**
- **285ml/10fl oz carton half-fat whipping cream, whipped**
- **395g/14oz strawberries, sliced**

1 Put half the biscuits into the bottom of a large, shallow dessert dish, or into six individual glass serving dishes.
2 Cover this with a thin layer of cream.
3 Arrange half the strawberries on top of the cream.
4 Repeat steps 1–3. Chill and serve.

Healthy Eating Notes

Try to base dessert dishes on fresh fruit. Cut down on fat and calories by choosing half-fat cream, virtually fat-free fromage frais or low-fat natural yoghurt.

Speedy Trifle

A kids' favourite and one of those desserts that can be made in advance, this recipe makes use of an instant custard mix so there's no need to worry about disguising those lumps. You can choose any fruit, but remember to buy the fruit canned in natural juice or fruit juice, rather than in syrup. If you have more time, you may want to make a sugar-free jelly and pour this over the fruit. Allow it to set in the refrigerator for about 45 minutes, then add the custard and cream.

Preparation time: 25 minutes
Serves: 6

- 415g/14¹/₂oz can fruit cocktail in natural juice
- 8 trifle sponge fingers or 4 trifle sponges (approx. 115g/4oz)
- 70g/2¹/₂oz packet low-fat instant custard mix
- 140ml/5fl oz/²/₃ cup half-fat whipping cream
- 2 kiwi fruits, sliced

1 Drain the fruit juice from the fruit cocktail and set aside.
2 Arrange the drained fruit and sponge cake in the bottom of a large pudding bowl.
3 Pour the reserved fruit juice over the sponge cake. Place the bowl in the refrigerator to chill.
4 Meanwhile, make up the custard with boiling water as indicated on the packet. Allow to cool.
5 Pour the custard over the sponge and fruit mixture, and put the bowl back into the refrigerator.
6 Whip the cream and spread it over the chilled custard.
7 Decorate with the kiwi fruit and serve chilled.

Healthy Eating Notes

Standard trifle ingredients have been replaced with lower-fat and reduced-sugar versions by incorporating low-fat custard, canned fruit in natural juice and half-fat cream.

Pears in Blackcurrant Sauce

Fruit-based puddings are generally healthier choices for everyone. Here's a delicious speedy alternative to the usual pears in red wine. To save time, you can use canned pear halves in natural juice and omit step 1.

Preparation and cooking time: 15 minutes
Serves: 4

- **2 firm dessert pears, peeled, halved and cored**
- **1 piece stem ginger, quartered (optional)**
- **A few drops of lemon juice**
- **$1/_2$ tsp cornflour (cornstarch)**
- **2 tbsp (about 30g/1oz) reduced-sugar blackcurrant jam**

1 Put the pears, ginger (if used) and lemon juice into a pan with 140ml/5fl oz/$^2/_3$ cup of boiling water. Bring back to the boil, cover and simmer gently for about 10 minutes until the pears are cooked.
2 Meanwhile, mix the cornflour (cornstarch) into a paste with a little cold water. Heat the jam gently with 60ml/2fl oz/$^1/_4$ cup of water and the cornflour paste. Bring this slowly to the boil while stirring, and allow to thicken. Remove from the heat.
3 Arrange the pears, curved side up, on a serving dish. Pour the sauce over the pears and serve chilled.

Healthy Eating Notes

Look out for reduced-sugar jam and canned pears in natural juice to cut down on sweetness and sugar.

Apricot Rice Pudding

Traditional baked rice puds can take an hour or more to cook in the oven. Make use of this short-cut recipe which uses a can of ready-made low-fat rice pudding.

Preparation and cooking time: 15 minutes
Serves: 4

- **30g/1oz ready-to-eat dried apricots, chopped**
- **1 apple, peeled, cored and chopped**
- **1 cinnamon stick**
- **Pinch of nutmeg**
- **425g/15oz can low-fat rice pudding**

1 Place the apricots, apple, cinnamon and nutmeg in a pan with 140ml/5fl oz/$^2/_3$ cup boiling water. Bring back to the boil, cover and simmer till the apple is soft (about 5 minutes).
2 Add the rice pudding and mix well. Serve hot or chilled.

Healthy Eating Notes

If you have a poor appetite, a milk pudding can be a nourishing addition to your meals.

Further Support and Information

Diabetes UK (formerly the British Diabetic Association)
10 Parkway
London
NW1 7AA
Tel: 020 7424 1000
Fax: 020 7424 1001
Email: info@diabetes.org.uk
Website: www.diabetes.org.uk
Diabetes UK Careline: 020 7424 1030

Other Useful Websites

www.thinkwelltobewell.com
www.diabeteswellnessnet.org.uk
www.bda.uk.com

Books

Govindji, Azmina and Myers, Jill. *Diabetes, Recipes for Health*, Thorsons, 1995
Govindji, Azmina. *Great Healthy Food: Diabetes*, Carroll & Brown, 2001
Govindji, Azmina and Puddefoot, Nina. *Think Well To Be Well*, Diabetes Research & Wellness Foundation, 2002
Leeds, Dr Anthony, Brand Miller, Prof. Jennie, Foster-Powell, Kaye and Colagiuri, Dr Stephen. *The New Glucose Revolution* (formerly *The GI Factor*), Hodder & Stoughton, 2003

Index